INDEX

FIRST AID AT WORK

First Aid at Work

including Paediatric Basic Life Support and AED

Subject	Section	Page
Contents		01
First Aid at Work qualification details	01	02
What is first aid?	02	03
Legislation	03	04
Responsibilities	04	07
Action in an emergency	05	09
Primary survey	06	10
Secondary assessment	07	11
The respiratory system	08	15
Resuscitation and AED	09	16
Disorders of respiration	10	23
Disorders of circulation	11	25
Wounds and bleeding	12	27
Seizures	13	30

Subject	Section	Page
Minor burns and scalds	14	32
Foreign objects	15	33
Primary survey - recap	16	34
Bones, joints and muscle injuries	17	35
Head and spinal injuries	18	39
Chest and abdominal injuries	19	42
Specialised burn injuries	20	45
Eye injuries	21	46
Poisoning	22	48
Anaphylaxis	23	51
Major illnesses	24	52
Effects of extreme heat and cold	25	56
Bites and stings	26	58

First Aid at Work is published by: **Nuco Training Ltd**

© All rights reserved. No part of this publication may be reproduced, stored in a retrieval system or transmitted in any form or by any means without written permission from Nuco Training Ltd.

This publication is supplied subject to the condition that it shall not, by any way of trade or otherwise, be lent, re-sold, hired out or otherwise circulated without the prior consent of Nuco Training Ltd.

FIRST AID AT WORK QUALIFICATION DETAILS

FIRST AID AT WORK QUALIFICATION DETAILS

3-Day First Aid at Work

You must attend and successfully complete a 3-Day First Aid at Work Course to qualify as a First Aider in the workplace. The qualification is valid for a 3 year period from your achievement date (subject to assessment).

The course is run over a minimum of three days and should contain at least 18 contact hours. However, it is acceptable to run the course over a longer period, not exceeding 10 weeks, where each session lasts at least two hours.

2-Day FAW requalification

In order to requalify as a First Aider in the workplace, you must attend and successfully complete a 2-Day requalification course.

Employers need to arrange retraining before certificates expire. If the First Aider does not retrain or requalify before the expiry date on their current certificate, they are no longer considered competent to act as a First Aider in the workplace.

The course should be run over a minimum of two days and contain at least 12 contact hours. However, it is acceptable to run the course over a longer period, not exceeding 7 weeks, where each session lasts at least two hours.

Assessment details

The summative assessments should determine your ability to act safely, promptly and effectively when an emergency occurs at work and to deal with a casualty who:
- **Is unresponsive**
- **Requires cardiopulmonary resuscitation (CPR)**
- **Is choking**
- **Is wounded and bleeding**

In addition, the learner will be questioned about their knowledge of a range of first aid conditions.

Refresher training

The HSE strongly recommends that First Aiders undertake annual refresher training during any three-year FAW certification period. Although not mandatory, this will help qualified First Aiders maintain their basic skills and keep up-to-date with any changes to first aid procedures.

WHAT IS FIRST AID?

First aid, as the term implies, is the initial treatment given to someone who is injured or sick, prior to professional medical assistance arriving and taking over from you.

As a First Aider, your priorities for the casualty fall into the following categories:

PRESERVE life
Providing treatment immediately and not waiting for professional help to sort it out for you.

ALLEVIATE suffering
Making the casualty more comfortable, reducing their pain levels and offering lots of care and attention.

PREVENT further illness or injury
Applying a secure sterile dressing on the injured part to control the blood loss and prevent the risk of infection, for example.

PROMOTE recovery
Treating the casualty for shock and ringing for an ambulance.

LEGISLATION

For some, you may have a responsibility in the workplace for first aid. Should this be the case then you must be aware of legislation that ensures employers provide a duty of care, along with first aid provision for their employees, non-employees and contractors visiting their premises.

THE HEALTH AND SAFETY AT WORK ACT 1974

Also abbreviated to *HASAWA, HSW 1974, HASWA*

The primary piece of legislation covering occupational health and safety in the United Kingdom. The Health and Safety Executive (and other enforcing authorities) are responsible for enforcing the Act.

The Act defines the fundamental structure for managing health and safety in the workplace and places legal duties on employers, employees, suppliers, contractors, the self-employed and other persons involved in workplace activities.

THE MANAGEMENT OF THE HEALTH AND SAFETY AT WORK REGULATIONS 1999

These regulations generally make more explicit what employers are required to do to manage health and safety under the Health and Safety at Work Act.

The main requirement is to carry out a risk assessment, to identify suitable measures to control the risks in your workplace. You only need to record the assessment if you have five or more employees.

The HSE has guidance on these Regulations referred to as 'Managing for Health and Safety (HSG65)'.

THE HEALTH AND SAFETY (FIRST AID) REGULATIONS 1981 (1982 IN NORTHERN IRELAND)

The Health and Safety (First-Aid) Regulations 1981 require employers to provide adequate and appropriate equipment, facilities and personnel to ensure their employees and others receive immediate attention if they are injured or taken ill at work.

FIRST AID AT WORK PROVISION

When deciding the first aid requirements for their business, employers should refer to the HSE's L74 Guidance on the First Aid Regulations.

It provides guidance on:

- **Managing the provision of first aid** (First aid kit, equipment, rooms etc)
- **Requirements and training for First Aiders**
- **Requirements for appointed persons**
- **Making employees aware of first aid arrangements**
- **First aid and the self-employed**
- **Cases where first aid regulations do not apply**

Such considerations could include:

- **Inexperienced workers or employees with disabilities**
- **Employees who travel a lot, work remotely or work alone**
- **Employees who work shifts or out of hours**
- **Premises spread out across buildings/floors**
- **Workplace remote from emergency medical services**
- **Employees working at sites occupied by other employers**
- **Planned and unplanned absences of First Aiders**
- **Members of the public who visit the workplace**

A full copy of the L74 guidance can be downloaded or purchased from the HSE's website.

FIRST AID AT WORK PROVISION

You should liaise with management and other First Aiders to ensure:

- **There is an adequate number of First Aiders in place**
- **Appropriate equipment, kits and facilities are available**
- **A system is in place for incident and accident reporting**

It is vital that a risk assessment of first aid needs is conducted to ensure the correct level of provision is made.

FIRST AID AT WORK

The following table will guide you in ensuring that you have sufficient numbers of trained first aid personnel at your place of work.

1. From your risk assessment, what degree of hazard is associated with your work activities	2. How many employees do you have?	3. What first aid personnel do you need?	4. What injuries and illnesses have previously occurred in your workplace	5. Have you taken account of the factors below that may affect your first aid provision?
Low-hazard eg offices, shops, libraries	Fewer than 25	At least **1 appointed person**	• Ensure any injuries or illness that may occur can be dealt with by the First Aider's you provide • Where First Aider's are shown to be unnecessary, there is still a possibility of an accident or sudden illness, so you may wish to consider providing qualified First Aider's	• Inexperienced workers or employees with disabilities or particular health problems • Employees who travel a lot, work remotely or work alone • Employees who work out-of-hours • Premises spread out across buildings/floors • Workplace remote from the emergency services • Employees working at sites occupied by other employers • Planned & unplanned absences of first-aider/appointed person • Members of the public who visit the workplace
	25 - 50	At least **1 EFAW** trained First Aider		
	More than 50	At least **1 FAW** trained First Aider for every 100 employed (or part thereof)		
Higher hazard eg light engineering and assembly work, food processing, warehousing, extensive work with dangerous machinery or sharp instruments, construction, chemical manufacture	Fewer than 5	At least **1 appointed person**		
	5 - 50	At least **1 EFAW** or **FAW** trained First Aider, depending on the type of injuries that may occur		
	More than 50	At least **1 FAW** trained First Aider for every 50 employed (or part thereof)		

Information supplied by Health & Safety Executive. The Health and Safety (First-Aid) Regulations 1981 L74 (Third edition 2013)

FIRST AID KITS

The minimum level of first aid equipment is a suitably stocked and properly identified first aid container.

Every employer should provide, for each work site, at least one first aid container supplied with a sufficient quantity of first aid materials.

There is no mandatory list of items to be included in a first aid container. The decision on what to provide will be influenced by the findings of the first aid needs assessment. As a guide, where work activities involve low hazards, a minimum stock of first aid items might be:

- A leaflet giving general guidance on first aid
- 20 individually wrapped sterile plasters (assorted sizes) *hypoallergenic plasters can be provided if necessary*
- Two sterile eye pads
- Four individually wrapped triangular bandages, preferably sterile
- Six safety pins
- Two large sterile individually wrapped un-medicated wound dressings
- Six medium-sized individually wrapped un-medicated wound dressings
- A pair of disposable gloves

This is a suggested contents list only.

The contents of first aid containers should be examined frequently and restocked soon after use.

It is recommended that tablets and medicines should not be kept in the first aid container.

PERSONAL PROTECTIVE EQUIPMENT (PPE)

Employers should supply adequate PPE stored near to the first aid supplies. Such equipment could include hand sanitiser, face masks, safety glasses, ear protection, hi-vis vests and flashlights. Employers should also advise First Aiders on what PPE should be worn in which circumstances, ensuring that the First Aider's safety is the priority.

ADDITIONAL FIRST AID MATERIALS AND EQUIPMENT

The needs assessment may indicate that additional materials and equipment are required, for example scissors, burns dressings and individually wrapped moist wipes. They may be kept in the first aid container if there is room, or stored separately. If mains tap water is not readily available for eye irrigation, at least one litre of sterile water in sealed, disposable containers should be provided.

First Aid at Work does not include giving tablets or medicines to treat illness, but you can assist an individual in taking it, if it is their own medication.

It is recommended that tablets and medicines should not be kept in the first aid container. However, the one exception is heart attacks. Therefore, for heart attack management, you can assist a casualty in taking one aspirin tablet (300mg) and ask them to chew it slowly, providing you are confident that the casualty is not allergic to it.

If you are in any doubt, then you **MUST NOT** administer it. Aspirin **MUST NOT** be administered to anyone under the age of 16.

LEGISLATION continued

ACCIDENT AND INCIDENT REPORTING

Irrespective of the severity of the accident or incident, it is vital that all such occurrences are reported and filed by the employer.

Anyone can complete the accident book, and this book must comply with Data Protection legislation. Online electronic reporting is an acceptable form of recording accidents and incidents as an alternative to the hand-written accident book.

The information that should be recorded includes:

- **The date, time and place of the incident**
- **Name and job of the injured or ill person**
- **Details of the injury/illness and what first aid was given**
- **What happened to the casualty immediately afterwards?** (e.g. went back to work, went home, went to hospital)
- **Name and signature of the person reporting the incident**

Where the incident is of a severe nature, then the employer must comply with RIDDOR 2013.

RIDDOR is the law that requires employers, and other people in control of work premises, to report and keep records of:

- **Work-related accidents which cause death**
- **Work-related accidents which cause certain serious injuries** (reportable injuries)
- **Diagnosed cases of certain industrial diseases**
- **Certain 'dangerous occurrences'** (incidents with the potential to cause harm)

Reporting certain incidents is a legal requirement. The report informs the enforcing authorities about deaths, injuries, occupational diseases and dangerous occurrences, so they can identify where and how risks arise, and whether they need to be investigated.

Please visit www.hse.gov.uk/riddor/ for full details of what is reportable.

> **Online electronic reporting is an acceptable form of recording accidents and incidents.**

RESPONSIBILITIES

FIRST AID AT WORK

A First Aider has a number of responsibilities when dealing with an incident which can be broken up into the following categories:
1. Arrival at the scene
2. Dealing with casualties
3. Casualty communication
4. Contacting the emergency services
5. Prioritise the first aid treatment
6. Clearing up process and infection control

1. ARRIVAL AT THE SCENE

Make the area safe and gather as much information about the incident as you can. The history of the incident and any casualty information about their illness or injury could help you decide your course of initial treatment.

A bystander can be of great benefit to you - don't be afraid to summon for help. A bystander can make a telephone call, get a first aid kit, return with the defibrillator, manage the crowd and traffic, and generally support you.

CONSENT

A responsive adult must agree to receive first aid treatment.

'**Expressed consent**' means that the casualty gives their permission to receive care and treatment. To obtain consent, first identify yourself, tell them about your level of training and ask if it's ok to help them.

'**Implied consent**' means that permission to perform first aid care on an unresponsive casualty is assumed. This is based on the idea that a reasonable person would give their permission to receive lifesaving treatment if they were able to.

When caring for vulnerable groups such as children and the elderly then consent must be gained from a parent, family member or legal guardian. When life-threatening situations exist and the parent, family member or legal guardian is not available, you must provide first aid care based on implied consent.

2. DEALING WITH CASUALTIES
- Prioritise your treatment, particularly if you have multiple casualties
- Ensure safety for all
- Protect against contamination
- Be calm and confident
- Ensure that the appropriate emergency services have been called for

3. CASUALTY COMMUNICATION
- Be honest about their condition, without exaggerating it
- Be careful of what you say which could distress them further
- Maintain eye contact when talking to them, and be aware of your body language
- Take your time when talking to them
- Allow your casualty to explain how they are feeling if they are able to
- In respect of their injury, avoid medical terms that they may not understand

SECTION 4 | PAGE 7

RESPONSIBILITIES continued

4. CONTACTING THE EMERGENCY SERVICES

As soon as you have identified the extent of the injury or illness, then it may be necessary to contact the emergency services. They can be contacted by dialling 999 or 112. Activate the speaker function on the phone to aid communication with the ambulance service.

They will also require specific details about the location of the incident. It is imperative that you have the full details of where you are, particularly if the premises are large and have multi-floors or other buildings to consider.

Only dial 999 if it is necessary and consider other services such as Police and Fire, dependent on the incident.

Remember **LIONEL** when making this call:

- **L** Location
- **I** Incident
- **O** Other services
- **N** Number of casualties
- **E** Extent of injuries
- **L** Location - repeat

5. PRIORITISE YOUR FIRST AID TREATMENT

- **Breathing** – deal with casualties who are not breathing normally first
- **Bleeding** – deal with any major bleeding and treat the casualty for shock
- **Burns/breaks** – treat burns and immobilise any bone injuries
- **Other conditions** – treat appropriately

Remember your priorities. Ensure that their airway remains open and that they are breathing normally for themselves.

Rescuers should take appropriate safety precautions where feasible, especially if the casualty is known to have a serious infection such as tuberculosis (TB), severe acute respiratory distress syndrome (SARS) or coronavirus (COVID-19).

During any outbreak of a highly infectious condition, protective precautions for the rescuer are essential.

6. THE CLEARING UP PROCESS AND INFECTION CONTROL

You must minimise the risk of infection from the outset when dealing with any incident. This applies to you, the casualty, and any bystanders. Similarly, when the casualty has been treated it is vital that all soiled dressings etc, are disposed of correctly.

- Wash your hands and wear disposable gloves
- Avoid coughing and sneezing over the wound, and avoid touching it
- Dispose of all soiled dressings, including gloves, in an appropriately marked *(orange/yellow)* plastic bag
- Dispose of sharp items, including syringes and needles, in a purpose made sharps bin and dispose of it appropriately. It may mean taking it to your local hospital for correct disposal

ACTION IN AN EMERGENCY

FIRST AID AT WORK

When confronted with any emergency situation, you need to take **SHAPE**!

S **SAFETY AND PROTECTION**
You must ensure the safety for all. Ensure you are adequately protected against the risk of infection and any other adverse element such as chemicals and gases

H **HAZARDS**
Be aware of potential hazards such as traffic, chemicals, fire, gas, electricity etc

A **ASSESS THE SITUATION**
Before rushing in to deal with an incident, you must assess the situation that you are confronted with

P **PRIORITISE**
Ensure you prioritise the injuries, particularly if you have multiple casualties

E **ENVIRONMENT**
Pay attention to the environment around you, and do not take risks. Jumping into water to save a drowning victim is not a good idea if you can't swim!

PRIMARY SURVEY

Irrespective of the incident you are confronted with, you must carry out an initial assessment of the situation including your casualty.

This is popularly known as the primary survey. The contents of this survey can be remembered easily by using the mnemonic **DR ABC**.

D — DANGERS
The area must be safe before you offer your casualty any treatment.
Safe for you primarily, not forgetting any bystanders and of course your casualty.

R — RESPONSE
Approach the casualty, ideally from their feet. This reduces the risk of the casualty hyper-extending their neck should they be responsive.

YOU CAN PERFORM A RESPONSIVE CHECK BY USING THE AVPU SCALE.

Alert - If they are fully responsive, then ascertain the extent of their injury and deal with it appropriately.

Voice - "Are you all right?"
If they are not alert, then see if they will respond to a voice command.

Place your hands on their shoulders and gently shake them.
If they don't respond to a voice command, then try shaking them gently by the shoulders.
NB: do not shake them if you suspect a spinal or head injury.

Unresponsive - If there is no response at all, they must be deemed as being unresponsive.

> The casualty who is **unresponsive and not breathing normally** is in cardiac arrest and requires CPR.
> Immediately following cardiac arrest blood flow to the brain is reduced to virtually zero, which may cause seizure-like episodes that may be confused with epilepsy.
> You should be suspicious of cardiac arrest with any casualty that presents seizure like symptoms and carefully assess whether they are breathing normally.

If your casualty responds, leave them in the position in which you find them providing there is no further danger. Try to find out what is wrong with them and treat accordingly. Call for professional medical help if it is needed and reassess them regularly.

If you are on your own, you should shout for help. Ideally you should never leave your casualty on their own.

A bystander can be a great benefit to you such as:

- Calling for an ambulance
- Fetching the first aid kit and defibrillator if you have one
- Helping you if they are trained to do so
- A support for you
- Managing crowds and hazards
- Consoling relatives and friends
- Cleaning up

A — AIRWAY
Turn the casualty onto their back and then open the airway using the head tilt and chin lift method:

- Place our hand on their forehead and gently tilt their head back
- With two fingertips under the point of their chin, lift the chin to open the airway
- Be careful not to press on the fleshy part under the chin as it could restrict the airway

Support their head in this position in order to perform a breathing check.

B — BREATHING
Look, listen and feel for normal breathing for no more than 10 seconds.

- **Look** for chest movement
- **Listen** at their mouth for breath sounds
- **Feel** for air on your cheek

In the first few minutes after cardiac arrest, a casualty may be barely breathing, or taking infrequent, noisy, gasps. This is often termed agonal breathing or gasping, and must not be confused with normal breathing. If you have any doubt whether breathing is normal, act as if it is not normal and prepare to commence CPR.

C — CPR FOR A NON-BREATHING CASUALTY
If your casualty **is not breathing normally**, then an ambulance must be summoned immediately. Lone rescuers should utilise the speaker function on their phone when making this call.
If you have a bystander at hand, ask them to make this important call so that you can commence cardiopulmonary resuscitation, or CPR without delay. (see page 16).

You can also ask your bystander to find and bring an Automated External Defibrillator (AED) to you, if one is available.

If your casualty is **breathing normally** and has no major physical trauma, they should be placed in the recovery position (see page 11) and an ambulance should be summoned.

If your casualty has sustained physical trauma, then the injuries should be treated accordingly and the casualty left in the position found. However, if you believe their airway is at risk, then the recovery position should be used.

Ensure that you monitor the casualty's breathing whilst waiting for the ambulance.

If you are unsure about the extent of the injury, then you should perform a top-to-toe survey (see page 13).

SECONDARY ASSESSMENT

CASUALTY ASSESSMENT

As soon as you have completed your primary survey, and you have established that your casualty is breathing normally, you must then move on to the secondary assessment in order to determine the extent of their injury or illness, irrespective of whether they are responsive or not.

In order to make a diagnosis of their condition, there are three key factors to consider:

HISTORY
- Ask your casualty or bystanders what happened
- Examine the environment for obvious signs relating to the incident
- Ask your casualty about their condition. Do they have their own medication? Has it happened before? Where does it hurt? How painful is it?
- Ask the casualty their name. Is there any family present that could answer the questions about their condition?

SIGNS
- What can you see in respect of the injury or condition?
- Use all your other senses. What can you smell, hear and feel?

SYMPTOMS
This is how the casualty will be feeling, ask them how they are feeling.
- Communication is very important to ascertain the extent of their injury/illness
- Continue to question their well-being throughout your assessment as they may have deteriorated which may influence your decision on the appropriate treatment

The recovery position

If your casualty is unresponsive, but breathing normally, with no evidence of major physical trauma, then your priority is to ensure that their airway is not compromised in any way and that it remains open. Rather than leaving them on their back or in a slumped position, an effective way of achieving this is to place them in the recovery position.

Whilst the casualty remains in this position, it will allow vomit to drain from the mouth and prevent them from rolling onto their back should you have to leave them.

1. Remove the casualty's glasses, if present
2. Kneel beside the casualty and make sure that both their legs are straight
3. Place the arm nearest to you out at a right angle to their body, elbow bent with the hand palm-up. Do not force the arm, let it fall naturally, but close to this position
4. Bring the far arm across the chest, and hold the back of the hand against their cheek nearest to you
5. Grab hold of the far leg with your other hand, and raise the knee so that their foot is kept to the floor. This will be your lever for rolling them over
6. Keeping their hand pressed against their cheek, pull on the far leg to roll them towards you onto their side with their head supported all the way
7. Tilt the head back to make sure that the airway remains open
8. If necessary, adjust the hand under their cheek to keep the head tilted and facing downwards to allow liquid material to drain from the mouth

SECTION 7 | PAGE 11

SECONDARY ASSESSMENT continued

9. Adjust the upper leg so that both the hip and knee are bent at right angles

10. Check breathing regularly

11. If you have a bystander available to you, then this is the time to send them to call for an ambulance ensuring they have all the appropriate information, and in particular, the condition of the casualty

12. If you have no bystander, you must call for an ambulance yourself

If they have to be kept in the recovery position for **more than 30 minutes** turn them to the opposite side to relieve the pressure on the lower arm.

You must continue to monitor their breathing whilst waiting for the emergency services to take over. If they stop breathing normally, then you must call the emergency services with an update and commence CPR immediately.

It will also be worth monitoring and noting other changes such as colouration of the skin, their temperature and responsiveness levels.

PREGNANT WOMEN
Always put an unresponsive pregnant woman in the recovery position on her **left side**. This prevents compression of the Inferior vena cava (large vein) by the uterus, which could be fatal for both the mother and the child.

SUSPECTED SPINAL INJURY
If you suspect a spinal injury and you cannot maintain an open airway in the position you found them, care must be taken in moving them.

Keep the casualty's back straight and support the head throughout.

It would be extremely useful to have help in moving the casualty.

The trained person should assume control when moving them.

Top-to-toe survey

If you are confident that your casualty has not sustained an injury, then place them in the recovery position and call for an ambulance. However, if you are unsure about the extent of the injury, then you should conduct a top-to-toe survey so that you can offer them appropriate treatment. As the term suggests, you should start at their head and work your way down to their feet.

You should wear gloves throughout this survey.

HEAD, FACE AND NECK
Ensure that the airway is clear and that there are no visible obstructions.

Look for bleeding, or any loss of fluids from the ears, eyes, nose and mouth. Feel for bumps, indentations and swelling around the head. Smell for unusual odour on the breath. Look for abnormal skin colouring and feel for it's temperature.

CHEST AND SHOULDERS
Check the collarbones for any fracture or deformity. Check the casualty's face for a response if you do suspect anything abnormal whilst assessing.

Again, gently squeeze the rib-cage for anything abnormal and check for a response. Look at the rise and fall of the chest for abnormal breathing.

SPINE
Get your hands behind your casualty and feel the top and base of the spine for abnormalities, and any other evidence of trauma.

Look at the position of how your casualty is laying. If you suspect a spinal injury, then support them in the position found, maintain an open airway and summon an ambulance immediately. If you are unable to maintain an open airway, then you must carefully place them in the recovery position.

ABDOMEN
Assess for any obvious signs of trauma such as blood loss. Very carefully press down on the abdominal area feeling for bumps and firmness and looking for bruising. Observe your casualty for a response when making this assessment.

PELVIS
Do not squeeze or rock the pelvis as it could complicate any potential injury.

Look for evidence of incontinence and bleeding and how the legs are laying. Look to see if the legs are splayed, or if one leg appears shorter than the other.

ARMS
Check each arm for obvious signs of trauma including blood loss and swelling.

Check for needle marks. See if the casualty is wearing an identity bracelet that may tell you of any condition they may have such as diabetes, anaphylaxis etc.

Check the hands for bruising and disfigurement.

Check for needle marks between the fingers.

LEGS AND EXTREMITIES
Check each leg and foot for obvious signs of trauma including blood loss and swelling. If you suspect a fracture, then it is imperative that you immobilise the limb and prevent any movement. Check the ankles for bruising and possible needle marks.

When you have completed this survey, now is the time to call for an ambulance ensuring that they are aware of any injury, as well the extent of it.

Your priority as a First Aider is to maintain an open airway for your casualty. If the casualty has no major physical trauma, then you must place them in the recovery position and monitor them whilst waiting for the ambulance to arrive.

If the airway is compromised in any way then, irrespective of the injury, the casualty must be placed in the recovery position.

SECONDARY ASSESSMENT continued

OBSERVATION CHART

The information from this chart will be very valuable when decisions are taken about further treatment

- Tick the appropriate boxes and update them at ten-minute intervals
- Send the completed chart and any notes with the casualty when he or she leaves your care

DATE .... / .... / ....   CASUALTY'S NAME ....

Time of observation (10-minute intervals)			0	10	20	30	40	50
EYES	Open spontaneously	4						
Observe for reaction	Open to speech	3						
while testing other responses	Open to painful stimulus	2						
	No response	1						
MOVEMENT	Obeys commands	6						
Apply painful stimulus:	Points to pain	5						
pinch the ear lobe or	Response to painful stimulus	4						
skin on back of hand	Bends in response to pain	3						
	Stretches in response to pain	2						
	No response	1						
SPEECH	Responds sensibly to questions	5						
When testing responses,	Seems confused	4						
speak clearly and directly,	Uses inappropriate words	3						
close to casualty's ear	Incomprehensible sounds	2						
	No response	1						
	TOTAL SCORE							

PULSE (Beats per minute)

Take pulse at wrist or neck on adult; inner arm on baby

Note the rate / beats	
Weak = W	
Regular = R	
Strong = S	

	0	10	20	30	40	50
Over 110						
101-110						
91-100						
81-90						
71-80						
61-70						
Below 61						

BREATHING (breaths per minute)

Note rate / quality:	
Quiet = Q	
Noisy = N	
Difficult = DIFF	
Easy = E	

	0	10	20	30	40	50
Over 40						
31-40						
21-30						
11-20						
Below 11						

THE RESPIRATORY SYSTEM

Our ability to breathe is thanks to our respiratory system which is made up primarily of our airways and our lungs.

We are able to breathe in and out spontaneously providing we have air to breathe and the airways are open.

Air breathed in
- Nitrogen - 78%
- Oxygen - 21%
- Argon and other gases - 1%

COMPOSITION OF AIR

When we breathe in the diaphragm contracts and flattens, the ribs are elevated, and as negative pressure is produced in the chest cavity, there is increased pressure in the abdomen. This draws air into the lungs to equalise the pressure.

We exhale when the diaphragm relaxes and the chest wall and lung tissue returns to their original size.

Respiration is achieved through the mouth, nose, trachea, lungs, and diaphragm. Oxygen enters the respiratory system through the mouth and the nose. The oxygen then passes through the larynx (where speech sounds are produced) and the trachea which is a tube that enters the chest cavity. In the chest cavity, the trachea splits into two smaller tubes called the bronchi. Each bronchus then divides again forming the bronchioles. These bronchial tubes lead directly into the lungs where they divide into many smaller tubes which connect to tiny sacs called alveoli. The average adult's lungs contain about 600 million of these spongy, air-filled sacs that are surrounded by capillaries. The inhaled oxygen passes into the alveoli and then enters the capillaries (diffusion) into the arterial blood which is taken back to the heart for circulating around the body.

Meanwhile, the waste-rich blood from the veins releases its carbon dioxide into the alveoli. The carbon dioxide follows the same path out of the lungs when you breathe out.

Approximately 25% of the available oxygen in each breath is used, as our body can only cope with so much each time we breathe in.

Carbon dioxide and other non-essential gases are breathed out and the whole process is repeated between 10 – 20 times per minute for an average adult.

The Respiratory System

Labels: Pharynx (throat), Larynx (voicebox), Oesophagus, Trachea (windpipe), Bronchi, Right lung, Nasal cavity, Mouth, Epiglottis, Left lung, Alveoli (air sacs), Bronchioles (small airways), Pleura, Diaphragm

RESUSCITATION AND AED

PRINCIPLES OF RESUSCITATION

Cardiopulmonary resuscitation (CPR) is an emergency procedure which is attempted in an effort to return life to a person who is not breathing normally for themselves.

This procedure combines chest compressions with rescue breaths. The chest compression replaces the heart's ability to pump oxygenated blood around the body, particularly to the vital organs such as the brain.

Rescue breathing provides the casualty, who is unable to breathe normally for themselves, valuable oxygen that is transported around the body by the chest compressions.

Without oxygen, brain damage can occur within three minutes. Therefore, your immediate action is paramount.

Referring back to Primary Survey, i.e. DR ABC, then you will have established that your casualty is not breathing normally.

Your immediate action now is to contact the emergency services and ask for an ambulance, ensuring that you state that your casualty is not breathing normally.

If you have a bystander at hand, then send them to make this important call. You can also ask your bystander to find and bring an Automated External Defibrillator (AED) to you, if one is available.

However, if you are on your own, then you **must** call the emergency services yourself. Stay with the casualty when making this call if possible.

If you are able to, activate the speaker function on your phone to aid communication between you and the emergency services.

Commence CPR without delay.

1. START WITH 30 CHEST COMPRESSIONS

- **Kneel by the side of your casualty**
- **Place the heel of one hand in the centre of the casualty's chest** (which is the lower half of the casualty's breastbone (sternum)

- Place the heel of your other hand on top of the first hand
- Interlock the fingers of your hands and ensure that pressure is not applied over their ribs. Do not apply any pressure over the upper abdomen or the bottom end of the sternum
- Position yourself vertically above their chest and, with your arms straight, press down on the sternum approximately 5cm (but not more than 6cm)

- After each compression, release all the pressure on the chest without losing contact between your hands and the sternum Do not lean on the chest.
- Repeat 30 chest compressions at a speed of 100 - 120 compressions per minute with as few interruptions as possible
- Compression and release should take an equal amount of time

In most circumstances it will be possible to identify the correct hand position for chest compressions, without removing the casualty's clothes. If you are in any doubt, then remove outer clothing.

2. GIVE 2 RESCUE BREATHS
After 30 chest compressions open the airway again using head tilt and chin lift.

- Pinch the soft part of their nose closed, using the index finger and thumb of your hand on their forehead
- Allow their mouth to open, but maintain chin lift
- Take a normal breath and place your lips around their mouth, making sure that you have a good seal
- Blow steadily into their mouth whilst watching for their chest to rise, taking about one second as in normal breathing; this is an effective rescue breath

- Maintaining head tilt and chin lift, watch for their chest to fall as air comes out
- Take another normal breath and blow into the casualty's mouth once more to achieve a total of two effective rescue breaths. Do not interrupt compressions by more than 10 seconds to deliver two breaths. Then return your hands without delay to the correct position on the sternum and give a further 30 chest compressions

If the initial rescue breath of each sequence does not make the chest rise as in normal breathing, then, before your next attempt:
- Check the casualty's mouth and remove any visible obstruction
- Re-check that there is adequate head tilt and chin lift
- Do not attempt more than two breaths each time before returning to chest compressions

In order to reduce the risk of cross-contamination, there are various protective shields and masks available that will significantly reduce this risk. For more information about infection control please see page 8.

Repeat 30 compressions and 2 breaths until
- A health professional tells you to stop
- The casualty is definitely waking up, moving, opening their eyes and breathing normally
- You become exhausted

It is rare for CPR alone to restart the heart. Unless you are certain the casualty has recovered, continue with CPR.

Signs the casualty has recovered include:
- Waking up
- Moving
- Opens eyes

AND
- They start breathing normally again

Be prepared to restart CPR immediately if the casualty deteriorates.

It must be emphasised that if you are unable to give rescue breaths for whatever reason, then you must continue with chest-compression-only CPR.

If there is more than one rescuer present, another should take over CPR about every 1-2 minutes to prevent fatigue.

Ensure the minimum of delay during the changeover of rescuers and do not interrupt chest compressions.

IF YOU HAVE ACCESS TO AN AED

As soon as it arrives, switch it on and attach the electrode pads on the casualty's chest. Follow the voice prompts. If more than one rescuer is present, CPR should be continued whilst the electrode pads are being attached to the chest.

(See pages 18 to 20 for AED use)

RESUSCITATION AND AED continued

THE CHAIN OF SURVIVAL

It is critical that you follow this chain when you are dealing with a casualty who is not breathing normally.

Early recognition and call for help
Recognise those at risk of cardiac arrest, and call for help in the hope that early treatment can prevent arrest.

Early CPR
Start CPR to buy time until medical help arrives.

Early defibrillation
Defibrillators give an electric shock to re-organise the rhythm of the heart.

Defibrillation within 3-5 minutes of cardiac arrest can produce survival rates as high as 50-70%.

Each minute of delay to defibrillation reduces the probability of survival to hospital discharge by 10%.

Post-resuscitation care
Provide professional help in order to restore the quality of life.

DEFIBRILLATION USING AN AED

When the AED arrives, you must immediately unpack it and prepare to fix the pads to the casualty. If you have trained help, then allow them to continue with CPR until you are ready. If not, then stop CPR and unpack it yourself.

If your casualty is wearing a wired bra, then this must be removed or cut through to expose the chest, particularly the area where the pads are to be fixed. Similarly, if your casualty is wearing jewellery that may come into contact with the pads, then it must be removed.

The majority of pads will be clearly marked on where they should be fixed. Depending on the make and model of the AED, the pads will generally come as two separate pads. Some will come as a single pad. Ensure that the film that is protecting the sticky pads is removed.

If your casualty has a pacemaker fitted, then ensure that the pads are placed at least 10cms away from it.

Do not place the pads directly on top of it. A pacemaker should be clearly identifiable, from a scar or what appears to be a small plate under the skin.

> **It may be necessary to prepare the casualty's chest in order for the pads to adhere. Do not waste valuable time shaving inappropriately.**

FIRST AID AT WORK

Most AED pads are labelled left and right, or carry a picture of the placement. It does not matter if these pads are reversed. What is important is that should they be placed the wrong way round, they must be left in place because the adhesive may well be removed or compromised if you swap them around.

In respect of switching the AED on, they will vary from one AED to another. Some will switch themselves on as soon as the lid is removed or opened. Others will have a button to press to switch it on.

It is important that you familiarise yourself with the AED you have.

All AED's will have a voice prompt and it is important that you follow these prompts.

Some AED's will also have a screen giving you the commands. This can be a very useful aid for those who are hard of hearing.

It is important from here on in to follow these prompts as soon as the pads are connected and the AED is switched on.

The AED will need to analyse the heart's rhythm. You will be prompted to ensure that no-one is touching the casualty, including yourself. Anyone touching the casualty could have an adverse effect on detecting the correct rhythm of your casualty's heart.

Dependent on the model you have, analysis will automatically happen, or you may have to push the 'Analyse' button.

You have to take control of the situation and move people away from the casualty.

Your next prompt could be to shock the casualty. Your AED may do this automatically, or you may have to press the 'Shock' button.

Again, manage the situation and ensure that no-one is touching the casualty.

Keep following the prompts from the AED.

If you are prompted to commence CPR, then quality CPR is important.

In essence you must continue with CPR until the AED tells you to stop to either analyse the casualty's heart rhythm, or it decides that a shock should be given.

Ensure that you compress at the right depth (5-6cms) and at the right speed (100-120 chest compressions per minute).

Under the current Resuscitation guidelines, you will be administering CPR for two minutes before the AED will prompt you to stop in order for it to analyse the heart's rhythm.

SECTION 9 | PAGE 19

RESUSCITATION AND AED continued

You must continue to follow the prompts until professional medical help takes over from you, your casualty recovers, or you become too exhausted to continue. Recovery will mean that your casualty shows signs of regaining responsiveness, such as coughing, opening their eyes, speaking or moving purposefully AND they start to breathe normally for themselves. To ensure they are breathing normally, conduct a breathing check.

If you are confident that they are breathing normally, place them in the recovery position with the pads attached and connected to the AED.

You must continue to monitor their breathing until professional medical help arrives and takes over from you.

ADULT BASIC LIFE SUPPORT

CHECK FOR DANGERS → **CHECK FOR A RESPONSE** → **YES**: If responsive, check for injuries and treat accordingly. Call the emergency services if required.

NO → If you are on your own, you should shout for help. Ideally you should never leave your casualty on their own.

↓

OPEN THE AIRWAY → Use minimum head tilt and lift the chin carefully.

↓

Check for normal breathing for no more than 10 seconds. → **YES**: If breathing normally, check for any injuries and place them in the recovery position if no major trauma is found. Call the emergency services and monitor their breathing.

NO ↓

If help is available, send them to call the emergency services and to bring a defibrillator back with them if one is available. → **NO**: If no help is available you must call them yourself and return with a defibrillator if one is available.

YES ↓

Give 30 chest compressions followed by 2 breaths.

↓

Continue with CPR until the casualty recovers, the emergency services take over or you become exhausted.

NB: If a defibrillator is available, then connect it immediately to the casualty and follow the voice prompts. If you have trained help available, then they can start CPR whilst you are preparing the casualty for defibrillation. **(See pages 18 to 20 for AED use)**

PAGE 20 | SECTION 9

PAEDIATRIC RESUSCITATION

The term paediatric refers to children and infants (babies). A child is deemed as being aged 1 year old through to 18 years old, and an infant being aged under 1 year old.

If you are in any doubt regarding the age of the child, then treat them as an adult, as little harm will come to them by adopting the adult protocols.

As with any incident, you must carry out a primary survey.
The contents of this survey can be remembered easily by using the mnemonic **DR ABC**.

D DANGERS
Make sure the area is safe

R RESPONSE
Check for a response.

If they are responsive by answering or moving;
- Leave the child in the position in which you find them (provided they is not in further danger)
- Check their condition and get help if needed
- Reassess their condition regularly

If they are not responsive, then:
- Shout for help
- Turn them on to their back
- Gently stimulate the child and ask loudly, 'Are you all right?'
- An infant can be stimulated by rubbing the soles of their feet with your finger
- Do not shake infants, or children with suspected cervical spine injuries
- Use their name when talking to them

A AIRWAY
Open their airway using the head tilt and chin lift manoeuvre:
- Place your hand on their forehead and gently tilt their head back. Be very careful not to over extend this movement with an infant
- With two fingertips under the point of their chin, lift the child's chin. Use one finger for an infant. In either case, do not push on the soft tissues under the chin as this may block the airway.

B BREATHING
Look, listen and feel for normal breathing for no more than 10 seconds.

C CPR for a non-breathing casualty
For CPR on an infant see Page 21
For CPR on a child see Page 22

If they are breathing normally:
- Treat any injuries accordingly and put them in the recovery position
- Call for an ambulance if the injuries or condition requires it
- Continue to monitor their breathing

CHILD RECOVERY POSITION

INFANT RECOVERY POSITION

CPR FOR AN INFANT

IF YOU HAVE HELP AVAILABLE ask them to call for an ambulance immediately and to bring back an AED if they can find one.

The following modifications to the adult sequence will make it more suitable for use in infants:
- Carefully remove any obvious airway obstructions
- Give 5 initial rescue breaths

Take a breath and cover the mouth and nose of the infant with your mouth, making sure you have a good seal. If both the nose and mouth cannot be covered in the older infant, then attempt to seal only the infant's nose or mouth with your mouth (if the nose is used, close the lips to prevent air escape and vice versa).

IF YOU ARE ON YOUR OWN, perform CPR for 1 minute i.e. approximately 2 cycles of 30 chest compressions followed by 2 rescue breaths.

You must then call 999 for an ambulance yourself.

TECHNIQUE FOR GIVING CHEST COMPRESSIONS FOR AN INFANT
- Compress the chest by at least one-third of its depth which is approximately 4cm for an infant
- Use the tips of 2 fingers to compress the chest
- The compression rate should be between 100–120 per minute

Continue with CPR (30:2) until the emergency services take over from you, your casualty recovers* or you become too exhausted to continue.

Should an AED arrive, unpack it and connect it to your casualty. Follow the voice prompts.

* Recovery means that they start to show signs of life i.e. they wake up, or start moving, or open their eyes **and** they start to breathe normally for themselves.

2 FINGER CHEST COMPRESSIONS

SECTION 9 | PAGE 21

RESUSCITATION AND AED continued

CPR FOR A CHILD

IF YOU HAVE HELP AVAILABLE ask them to call for an ambulance immediately and to bring back an AED if they can find one.

The following modifications to the adult sequence will make it more suitable for use in children:

- Carefully remove any obvious airway obstructions
- Give 5 initial rescue breaths

IF YOU ARE ON YOUR OWN, perform CPR for 1 minute i.e. approximately 2 cycles of 30 chest compressions followed by 2 rescue breaths.

You must then call 999 for an ambulance yourself.

TECHNIQUE FOR GIVING CHEST COMPRESSIONS FOR A CHILD

- Compress the chest by at least one-third of its depth which is approximately 5cm for a child
- Use one or two hands for a child over 1 year to achieve an adequate depth of compression
- The compression rate should be between 100–120 per minute

Continue with CPR (30:2) until the emergency services take over from you, your casualty recovers* or you become too exhausted to continue.

Should an AED arrive, unpack it and connect it to your casualty. Follow the voice prompts.

*Recovery means that they start to show signs of life i.e. they wake up, or start moving, or open their eyes **and** they start to breathe normally for themselves.

DROWNING

Drowning is defined as respiratory impairment from being in, or under a liquid, normally water.

Drowning begins as a result of the casualty not being able to breathe because the airways are submerged below the surface of the liquid.

As with any incident, follow the **DR ABC** Primary Survey protocol:

D DANGERS
Consider the risk to yourself before attempting to rescue the casualty.
It may well be that chemicals are involved causing an additional toxic risk e.g. a slurry tank.

R RESPONSE
Check for a response as you would normally do.

A AIRWAY
Open the airway

B BREATHING
Check to see if they are breathing normally.

C CPR
If they are not breathing normally, shout for help and call 999 unless you have help at hand and then send them to make the call and to find an AED.

CPR PROCEDURE
- Call 999
- Open the airway
- Give 5 initial rescue breaths
- Follow with 30 chest compressions
- Repeat 2 rescue breaths followed by 30 chest compressions until the casualty recovers, or the emergency services take over from you
- Attach the AED when it arrives and follow the voice prompts. Ensure there is no direct contact with the casualty and the water when defibrillating

Many casualties that drown will regurgitate their stomach contents. If this is the case, roll them on to their side so that it drains out leaving a clear and open airway.

If the casualty recovers, place them in the recovery position, keep them warm and continue to monitor them.

PAGE 22 | SECTION 9

DISORDERS OF RESPIRATION

CHOKING - RESPONSIVE CASUALTY

There are many factors that can contribute to a respiratory disorder, including asthma, hypoxia, smoke inhalation and choking.

Choking is probably the most common of the disorders and probably the most distressing to suffer and to deal with.

Your immediate treatment is required. Should your casualty become unresponsive as a result of choking, then you will have to start resuscitation. You should suspect choking if someone is unable to speak or talk, particularly if they're eating.

Recognition of someone choking
- Difficulty in speaking and breathing
- Coughing or gagging
- Clutching at the throat and pointing to the mouth
- Pale, grey/blue skin tone in the later stages (cyanosis)
- Ultimately – unresponsiveness

If your casualty shows signs of a mild or partial airway obstruction then:
- Encourage them to cough
- Stay calm and offer plenty of encouragement and reassurance

If coughing becomes ineffective then provide treatment for a severe airway obstruction for an adult:
- Check their mouth and remove any obvious obstruction

Bend them forward and give up to five back blows

- Stand to the side and slightly behind your casualty
- Support the chest with one hand and lean them forward so that when the obstructing object is dislodged it comes out of the mouth rather than to go further down the airway
- Give up to five sharp blows between their shoulder blades with the heel of your other hand

Check to see if each back blow has relieved the airway obstruction.
The aim is to relieve the obstruction with each blow rather than to give all five unnecessarily.
Continued on page 24.

DISORDERS OF RESPIRATION continued

Give them up to five abdominal thrusts
- Stand behind your casualty and put both arms round the upper part of their abdomen

- Lean them forward
- Clench your fist and place it between the umbilicus (navel) **and the bottom end of their sternum** (breastbone)

- Grasp this hand with your other hand and pull sharply inwards and upwards
- Repeat up to five times

- Check to see if each abdominal thrust has relieved the airway obstruction. The aim is to relieve the obstruction with each thrust rather than to give all five unnecessarily
- If you have performed abdominal thrusts on a casualty, they must be sent to hospital to be examined for any internal injuries.

If the obstruction cannot be removed after the first cycle of back blows and abdominal thrusts, then you must call for an ambulance immediately.

Repeat the process of up to five back blows followed by up to five abdominal thrusts until the casualty recovers, or the emergency medical services take over from you.

If your casualty becomes unresponsive, then help them to the floor onto their back, call 999/112 and commence CPR immediately.

Before each rescue breath attempt, check in the mouth for any visible obstruction that can be removed easily without having to sweep the mouth with your fingers.

DISORDERS OF CIRCULATION

FIRST AID AT WORK

The circulatory system is our body's transport system for two fluids, namely, blood and lymph.

For the purposes of first aid we will focus on the transport of blood, also known as the cardiovascular system.

This system consists of the heart and blood vessels, which supply our body, and in particular, our vital organs such as the brain and heart, with blood containing oxygen and nutrients to keep them healthy.

Our heart is a hollow muscular pump, about the size of your fist, with two pairs of chambers. These chambers collect blood flowing back from our body after depositing the oxygen and nutrients, before being pumped back to the lungs to collect more oxygen so that the cycle of transportation can continue.

The adult heart beats approximately 60 – 80 times every minute and pumps approximately six litres of blood around our body every minute.

- Blood returning from the upper body
- Blood to lungs
- Oxygenated blood from lungs
- Blood returning from lower body
- Oxygenated blood to upper body
- Blood to lungs
- Oxygenated blood from lungs
- Oxygenated blood to lower body

The blood vessels within this system are:
- **Arteries**
  Deliver oxygenated blood from the heart to the body, with the exception of the pulmonary artery which carries deoxygenated blood from the heart to the lungs
- **Veins**
  Carry the de-oxygenated blood back to the heart
- **Capillaries**
  Much smaller vessels that form a link between the arteries, veins and body tissue to allow the transfer of oxygen and nutrients to the body and the waste products to be removed

Blood is made up of:
- **Plasma**
  The fluid component of the blood of which 90% is water
- **Platelets**
  Help to block the blood flow by clotting
- **Red cells**
  Transport the oxygen via the haemoglobin
- **White cells**
  Manufacture antibodies and fight infection and bacteria

DISORDERS OF CIRCULATION continued

HYPOVOLAEMIC SHOCK

There are a number of reasons why this system could fail, including blood loss, failure of the heart, poor circulation, a fall in blood pressure and the lack of oxygen contained within the body.

Other conditions include poisoning, vomiting, infection, burns and injury to the spinal cord, but this is by no means the definitive list.

As a First Aider, there are a number of things we can do for our casualty such as to stop the bleeding and to take pressure off the heart. This will be covered later, but one of your main concerns should be that hypovolaemic shock will set in very quickly if you don't react quickly enough, and shock can be a killer!

Hypovolaemic shock is best described as a failure or collapse of the circulatory system when the arterial blood pressure is too low to provide an adequate blood supply to the tissues.

Signs and symptoms of hypovolaemic shock
- **Ashen coloured skin** (grey/blue)
- **Clammy and cold skin to touch**
- **Feeling of sickness and thirst**
- **Their breathing will be rapid and shallow**
- **Rapid, weak pulse**

Treatment of hypovolaemic shock
- Deal with the injury or condition
- Make them comfortable and lay them down
- Raise both legs providing it does not compromise their injuries further
- Keep them warm and maintain their response levels by talking to them
- Call for an ambulance
- Monitor their response and breathing
- Do not allow them to smoke, eat or drink as it may affect their well-being and it could compromise further treatment

FAINTING

Fainting is a sudden, usually temporary, brief loss of responsiveness generally caused by insufficient oxygen in the brain.

The signs and symptoms are the same as shock with the exception that the pulse rate is slower.

A casualty who has fainted will generally make a rapid recovery and feel fine very quickly.

TREATMENT FOR SOMEONE WHO FEELS FAINT
- Help them to the floor and lie them down
- Raise and support their legs
- Offer them plenty of fresh air
- Sit them up gradually
- Comfort and reassure them

TREATMENT FOR SOMEONE WHO HAS FAINTED

If a person faints and does not regain responsiveness within one or two minutes, you should put them into the recovery position, monitor their breathing and medical assistance should be sought.

WOUNDS AND BLEEDING

FIRST AID AT WORK

TYPES OF WOUNDS

A wound can be best described as a type of injury in which the skin is torn, cut or punctured (an open wound), or where a blunt force created a contusion (a bruise).

In first aid there are 6 types of wounds that you should be familiar with:

INCISION — Clean cut as with a knife blade

LACERATION — Rough tear as with barbed wire

ABRASION — Scrape as with a gravel rash

CONTUSION — A blunt blow causing bruising

PUNCTURE — A stabbing type wound

VELOCITY — Gunshot wound

When a blood vessel is torn or severed, blood loss and shock cause the blood pressure to fall and the injured vessels will contract at the site of injury.

Platelets and proteins come into contact with the injured site and plug the wound.

This clotting process begins within ten minutes if the loss of blood is brought under control.

BLEEDING IS CLASSIFIED BY THE TYPE OF BLOOD VESSEL THAT IS DAMAGED.

Arterial Pumps from the wound with the heartbeat

Venous Gushes from the wound or pools at the site

Capillary Oozing at the site of injury

Once you have completed your initial casualty assessment for prioritising your treatment, you must follow the guidelines for personal protection and hygiene control before you begin to treat the casualty for bleeding, see below and next page.

Treatment for the control of bleeding

- Put on disposable gloves
- Expose and examine the wound
- **Apply direct pressure with your fingers or palm, preferably over a sterile dressing or non-fluffy clean pad** (you can ask your casualty to apply this pressure)
- Elevate and support the injured part for wounds that are not catastrophic
- Help the casualty to lie down and raise the legs if you suspect shock
- Secure the dressing with a bandage large enough to cover the wound
- If blood seeps through this dressing, remove both the dressing and bandage and apply pressure to the bleed with a new dressing
- Secure the new dressing with a bandage once the bleeding is under control
- Support the injured limb with a sling or bandaging if appropriate, providing the casualty allows you to do so
- Monitor their response levels and call for an ambulance

CATASTROPHIC BLEEDING

If you are unable to stop the bleeding because of the severity, then you will need to apply direct pressure continually and then pack the wound with haemostatic dressings, or apply a tourniquet.

If you have neither, then you must continue to apply direct pressure and consider making an improvised tourniquet. It is imperative that you call for an ambulance immediately for a severe, or catastrophic bleed.

To summarise the treatment for catastrophic bleeding

- **Do** apply direct pressure to the wound
- **Do** use a haemostatic dressing or tourniquet
- **Do not** apply indirect pressure to proximal pressure points
- **Do not** elevate an extremity

Fortunately, the vast majority of businesses would never have to deal with a catastrophic bleed in a first aid situation at work. For most First Aiders, blood loss can be controlled by following the guidelines as detailed in the left hand column.

> It must be emphasised that further training is required for First Aiders in respect of using haemostatic dressings or tourniquets.
>
> Please speak to your training provider.

WOUNDS AND BLEEDING continued

EMBEDDED OBJECTS

If during your examination of the wound you see an embedded object such as a piece of glass, then you must leave it in place and dress around it. Your aim is to stop the bleeding, but care must be taken not to put any direct pressure on the embedded object.

- Check the wound for anything embedded
- Apply dressing and pressure to either side of the object
- Apply a larger sterile dressing over the top
- Secure the bandage
- Elevate the injured limb
- Treat for shock

BLEEDING FROM ORIFICES

Signs, symptoms and causes

Site	Appearance	Cause
Mouth	Bright red, frothy, coughed up.	Bleeding in the lungs.
	Vomited blood, red or dark reddish brown.	Bleeding in the stomach.
Ear	Fresh bright-red blood.	Injury to ear, perforated eardrum.
	Thin, watery blood.	Head injury.
Nose	Fresh bright red blood.	Ruptured blood vessel in nostril.
	Thin, watery blood.	Skull fracture.
Anus	Fresh bright-red blood.	Injury to anus or lower bowel.
	Black tarry, offensive smelling stool.	Injury to upper bowel.
Urethra	Urine with red or smoky appearance and occasional clots.	Bleeding from the bladder, kidneys.
Vagina	Either fresh or dark blood	Menstruation, miscarriage, disease or injury to the vagina or womb.

TREATMENT

- Treat the cause where possible using sterile dressings
- Treat the casualty for shock
- Monitor their condition, particularly their breathing
- Call 999/112 for an ambulance
- Lay them injured side down where possible
- Do not try to plug the wound, but cover it with a sterile dressing
- Offer them plenty of reassurance
- Pay attention to the casualty's modesty and dignity, particularly if they are bleeding from the anus or vagina

AMPUTATIONS

Any part of the body that has been severed will need immediate hospital treatment.

There is almost certain to be severe blood loss, and your aim as a First Aider is to control the bleeding, treat for shock and to protect and transport the amputated body part to hospital with the casualty.

Your prompt and effective treatment may just allow the amputated part to be stitched back successfully with micro-surgery.

Signs and symptoms

- Bleeding
- Shock
- Severe pain in the majority of cases
- An open wound
- Amputated body part

Treatment

- Ensure that the area is safe. Turn off machinery etc, that may have caused the accident
- Control the loss of blood by applying direct pressure with a sterile, non-fluffy dressing
- Treat the casualty for shock
- Reduce the risk of cross-infection by wearing gloves
- Call 999/112 for an ambulance
- Wrap the amputated part in plastic such as cling-film
- Wrap it further in a cloth
- Submerge the wrapped and protected part in ice. It is important that the severed part does not make direct contact with the ice. Mark the package clearly with the casualty's name and ensure that it is transported to hospital with the casualty
- Protect and maintain an open airway
- Monitor their breathing. Be prepared to resuscitate the casualty if they stop breathing normally

MINOR CUTS AND GRAZES

Cuts and grazes are some of the most common injuries.

Minor cuts and grazes (where only the surface layer of skin is cut or scraped off) may bleed and feel slightly painful, but the affected area will normally scab over and heal quickly.

However, if the cut is in an area that is constantly moving, such as your knee joint, it may take longer to heal.

Depending on how deep the cut is and where it is on your body, a scar may remain once the cut has healed.

Deeper cuts may damage important structures below the skin such as nerves, blood vessels or tendons.

However, grazes that remove the deeper layers of skin are rare.

Most cuts and grazes can be easily treated by cleaning them thoroughly and covering them with a plaster or dressing.

Please bear in mind that hypoallergenic plasters are available should your casualty have an allergy to ordinary plasters.

SEEK MEDICAL HELP IF ANY OF THE BELOW APPLY:

You think there is damage to deeper tissues: signs include numbness (indicating injury to a nerve), blood spurting from the wound or bleeding that does not stop after five minutes of continuous firm pressure.

The wound is at risk of becoming infected: for example, a cut has been contaminated with soil, faeces or a dirty blade, or fragments of material such as grit or glass which can be seen in the wound.

The wound has become infected: signs include swelling of the affected area, pus coming from the wound, redness spreading from the wound and increasing pain. The wound cannot be closed with a plaster, or it starts to open up when it moves.

The wound will create an unwelcome scar: for example, if it occurs on a prominent part of the casualty's face.

> **TETANUS IMMUNISATION**
> If the wound has been contaminated by dirt or soil, then it is advisable to ask the casualty about their history of tetanus immunisation.
> Advise to seek medical advice if:
> - They have never been immunised
> - If they are unsure about their history of injections

BRUISING

Bruises are bluish or purple-coloured patches that appear on the skin when tiny blood vessels (capillaries) break or burst underneath it.

The blood from the capillaries leak into the soft tissue under the skin causing the discolouration.

Over time this fades through shades of yellow or green.

Bruises often feel tender or swollen at first.

What causes bruising?

Bruising is caused by internal bleeding (under the skin) due to a person injuring themselves by, for example, falling over, walking into something or playing sports.

Some people are naturally more likely to bruise than others, for example, the elderly may bruise more easily because their skin is thinner and the tissue underneath is more fragile.

Treatment for bruises

Treat bruises, initially, by limiting the bleeding. You can do this by cooling the area with a cold compress (a flannel or cloth soaked in cold water) or an ice pack wrapped in a towel.

To make an ice pack, place ice cubes or a packet of frozen vegetables in a plastic bag and wrap them in a towel. Hold this over the affected area for at least 10 minutes.

Do not put the ice pack straight onto the skin as this will possibly cause further damage.

Most bruises will disappear after around two weeks.

If the bruise is still there after two weeks, you should recommend that your casualty see their GP.

Internal bruising

Bruises don't just happen under the skin - they can also happen deeper in the body's tissues, organs and bones.

While the bleeding isn't visible, the bruises can cause swelling and pain.

You should recommend that your casualty seeks medical attention, or call for an ambulance if you feel the injury is of a serious nature, particularly if they have been involved in an accident.

NOSEBLEEDS

A common injury that is caused generally by a direct blow or sneezing. However, high blood pressure can also cause a sudden bleed with little warning.

If the blood is watery, then it could suggest a head injury, therefore making the incident far more serious i.e. possible skull fracture.

Treatment

- **Sit the casualty down and lean them forward**
- **Ask them to pinch the soft part of the nose as they lean forward**
- **Apply this pressure for 10 minutes and then release slowly**
- **Ask them to avoid rubbing or blowing their nose**
- **If you are unable to stop the bleeding, ask them to repeat the pinching process for a further 10 minutes**
- **If the bleeding continues beyond 30 minutes then you will need to seek medical advice**

  If you suspect a head injury, then an ambulance must be summoned.

> If the casualty is feeling faint or nausea, you may consider sitting the casualty on the floor with their back supported. This could potentially prevent a fall.

SEIZURES

WHAT IS EPILEPSY?

Epilepsy is a condition that affects the brain. When someone has epilepsy, it means they have a tendency to have epileptic seizures.

Anyone can have a one-off seizure, but this doesn't always mean they have epilepsy. Epilepsy is usually only diagnosed if someone has had more than one seizure, and doctors think it is likely they could have more.

Epilepsy can start at any age and there are many different types. Some types of epilepsy last for a limited time and the person eventually stops having seizures. But for many people epilepsy is a life-long condition.

WHAT ARE EPILEPTIC SEIZURES?

A seizure happens when there is a sudden burst of intense electrical activity in the brain. This causes a temporary disruption to the way the brain normally works.

The result is an epileptic seizure.

There are many different types of seizure. What happens to someone during a seizure depends on which part of their brain is affected. During some types of seizure, the person may remain alert and aware of what's going on around them, and with other types they may lose awareness. They may have unusual sensations, feelings, or movements. Or they may go stiff, fall to the floor and jerk.

WHAT CAUSES EPILEPSY?

Possible causes of epilepsy include:
- **Stroke**
- **A brain infection, such as meningitis**
- **Severe head injury**
- **Problems during birth which caused the baby to get less oxygen**

But in over half of all people with epilepsy, doctors don't know what caused it. Some may have a family history of epilepsy, suggesting that they may have inherited it.

Tonic-clonic seizures are the type of seizure most people recognise.

Someone having a tonic-clonic seizure goes stiff, loses responsiveness, falls to the floor and begins to jerk or convulse. They may go blue around the mouth due to irregular breathing. Sometimes they may lose control of their bladder or bowels, and bite their tongue or the inside of their mouth.

HOW TO HELP IF YOU SEE SOMEONE HAVING A TONIC-CLONIC SEIZURE

Do:

- **Protect them from injury** (remove harmful objects from nearby)
- **Cushion their head**
- **Look for an epilepsy identity card or identity jewellery** – it may give you information about their seizures and what to do
- **Time how long the jerking lasts**
- **Aid breathing by gently placing them in the recovery position once the jerking has stopped**
- **Stay with the them until they are fully recovered**
- **Be calmly reassuring**

Don't:

- Restrain their movements
- Put anything in their mouth
- Try to move them unless they are in danger
- Give them anything to eat or drink until they are fully recovered
- Attempt to bring them round

Call for an ambulance if:

- You know it is their first seizure or
- The jerking continues for more than five minutes or
- They have one tonic-clonic seizure after another without regaining responsiveness between seizures or
- They are injured during the seizure or
- You believe they need urgent medical attention

FOCAL SEIZURES

This type of seizure can also be called a partial seizure. Someone having a focal seizure may not be aware of their surroundings or what they are doing. They may have unusual movements and behaviour such as plucking at their clothes, smacking their lips, swallowing repeatedly or wandering around.

How to help if you see someone having a focal seizure.

Do:

- **Guide them away from danger** (such as roads or open water)
- **Stay with them until recovery is complete**
- **Be calmly reassuring**
- **Explain anything that they may have missed**

Don't:

- Restrain them
- Act in a way that could frighten them, such as making abrupt movements or shouting at them
- Assume they are aware of what is happening, or what has happened
- Give them anything to eat or drink until they are fully recovered
- Attempt to bring them round

Call for an ambulance if:

- You know it is their first seizure or
- The seizure continues for more than five minutes or
- They are injured during the seizure or
- You believe they need urgent medical attention

MINOR BURNS AND SCALDS

Burns and scalds are among the most serious and painful of injuries. They can be caused by a number of factors including fire, water, electricity, oils, hot surfaces, steam, chemicals and radiation.

CLASSIFICATION OF BURNS

Superficial
The outer layer of skin is burnt causing redness, tenderness and inflammation.

Typical factors causing this would be sunburn or touching a hot iron.

The skin is not broken or blistered.

Partial thickness
The outer layer of the skin is burnt and broken causing blistering, swelling, pain and rawness.

Full thickness
All the layers of skin have been damaged causing the skin to look pale, charred and waxy with fatty deposits. There may also be damage to the nerves.

When to send a casualty to hospital
Every year in the UK, around 175,000 people attend hospital accident and emergency departments for burns injuries.

People who may be at greater risk from the effects of burns, such as children under five years of age and pregnant women, should seek medical attention after a burn or scald.

Assessing the extent of the burn
One quick way to estimate the surface area that has been burned is to compare it to the size of the palm of the casualty's hand, which is roughly equal to 1% of the body's total surface area.

For other groups, you must send them to hospital if:
- The burns affect the hands, feet, face and genital areas
- Full thickness burns
- Burns that extend around a limb
- All partial thickness burns larger than 1% of the body's surface. The casualty's hand represents about 1% on the body's surface
- All superficial burns that represent 5% of the body's surface
- Burns with a mixed pattern of depth

If you are in any doubt, then you should seek medical advice.

Treatment of burns
- Ensure the area is safe, particularly from the source that created the burn or scald
- Wear disposable gloves
- Cool the burn with running tap water for 20 minutes
- If it's possible, remove any watches or jewellery around the affected area
- Cover the burn with a suitable sterile dressing that is not fluffy. You can cover it with cling film if you have no appropriate dressing
- Treat the casualty for shock
- Monitor their condition throughout and call for an ambulance if it deteriorates
- Remove them to hospital if you consider it appropriate

You must not:
- Apply any form of cream, ointment or fat to the affected area
- Burst any blister that may form
- Apply any form of adhesive dressing
- Remove anything that is stuck to the affected area

NB: The biggest risk associated with bursting blisters is infection

FOREIGN OBJECTS

FIRST AID AT WORK

A foreign object in first aid terms, relates to an object of any size that enters the body through many of its orifices, or penetrates the skin and is embedded.

You have to make a decision on whether you can remove it without having to seek medical help.

If a common embedded object such as a splinter is partly exposed, then it is acceptable to remove it with tweezers. First aid tweezers generally come in a sterile package. Washing grit away, under running water, can also be a useful treatment. If this won't remove the object, then the wound should be dressed with a sterile dressing, without putting direct pressure on the object, and then to seek medical attention.

However, for other objects such as glass or a fishing hook, they must be left in place and you should not attempt to remove it. Dress the wound appropriately and seek medical advice.

The nose

- **Objects pushed up the nose may cause blockages or infection**
  Keep your casualty calm and reassure them.
- **Get the casualty to breathe through their mouth**
- **Do not attempt to remove the object**
- **Send the casualty to hospital**

The ears

If a foreign object enters the ear and becomes lodged, it can cause damage to the ear canal, the eardrum and in some cases, cause temporary deafness.

The object should be left in the ear, unless it's a living object such as an insect that could be removed by flooding the ear with tepid water. If this doesn't work, then you must seek medical advice.

If you need to seek medical advice:

- **Cover the ear with a sterile dressing, taking care not to put any direct pressure on the object**
- **Send the casualty to hospital**

Swallowed objects

Small objects are commonly swallowed by children. Many will enter the digestive system without choking the casualty, and leave the body in its natural way. However, you should seek medical attention irrespective. If you know that the object was sharp or toxic, then you must seek urgent medical attention.

If the object becomes stuck in the respiratory tract, then you should follow the choking procedure.

Some sharp objects may stick in the throat, such as fish bones or glass. If this is the case, then you must seek urgent medical attention as the airway could swell which would affect the casualty's ability to breathe normally.

SECTION 15 | PAGE 33

PRIMARY SURVEY RECAP

Irrespective of the incident you are confronted with, you must carry out an initial assessment of the situation including your casualty.

This is popularly known as the primary survey.
The contents of this survey can be remembered easily by using the mnemonic **DR ABC**.

D DANGERS

The area must be safe before you offer your casualty any treatment. Safe for you primarily, not forgetting any bystanders and of course your casualty.

Failing to do this could result in you having more casualties to deal with, which could include yourself!

R RESPONSE

Approach the casualty, ideally from their feet. This reduces the risk of the casualty hyper-extending their neck should they be responsive.

YOU CAN PERFORM A RESPONSIVE CHECK BY USING THE AVPU SCALE.

Alert   If they are fully responsive, then ascertain the extent of their injury and deal with it appropriately.

Voice - "Are you all right?"
If they are not alert, then see if they will respond to a voice command.

Place your hands on their shoulders and gently shake them.
If they don't respond to a voice command, then try shaking them gently by the shoulders. NB: do not shake them if you suspect a spinal or head injury.

Unresponsive
If there is no response at all, they must be deemed as being unresponsive.

If your casualty responds, leave them in the position in which you find them providing there is no further danger. Try to find out what is wrong with them and treat accordingly.

Call for professional medical help if it is needed and reassess them regularly.

If you are on your own, you should shout for help. Ideally you should never leave your casualty on their own.

A bystander can be a great benefit to you such as:
- Calling for an ambulance
- Managing crowds and hazards
- Fetching the first aid kit and defibrillator if you have one
- Consoling relatives and friends
- Helping you if they are trained to do so
- Cleaning up
- A support for you

A AIRWAY

Turn the casualty onto their back and then open the airway using the head tilt and chin lift method:
- Place your hand on their forehead and gently tilt their head back
- With two fingertips under the point of their chin, lift the chin to open the airway
- Be careful not to press on the fleshy part under the chin as it could restrict the airway

Support their head in this position in order to perform a breathing check.

B BREATHING

Look, listen and feel for normal breathing for no more than 10 seconds.

Look for chest movement
Listen at their mouth for breath sounds
Feel for air on your cheek

In the first few minutes after cardiac arrest, a casualty may be barely breathing, or taking infrequent, noisy, gasps. This is often termed agonal breathing or gasping, and must not be confused with normal breathing.

If you have any doubt whether breathing is normal, act as if it is **not** normal and prepare to commence CPR.

C CPR for a non-breathing casualty

If your casualty **is not breathing normally**, then an ambulance must be summoned immediately. Lone rescuers should utilise the speaker function on their phone when making this call. If you have a bystander at hand, ask them to make this important call so that you can commence cardiopulmonary resuscitation, or CPR without delay. (see page 16).

You can also ask your bystander to find and bring an Automated External Defibrillator (AED) to you, if one is available.

If your casualty is **breathing normally** and has no major physical trauma, they should be placed in the recovery position (see page 11) and an ambulance should be summoned.

If your casualty has sustained physical trauma, then the injuries should be treated accordingly and the casualty left in the position found. However, if you believe their airway is at risk, then the recovery position should be used.

Ensure that you monitor the casualty's breathing whilst waiting for the ambulance.

If you are unsure about the extent of the injury, then you should perform a top-to-toe survey (see page 13).

The casualty who is **unresponsive** and **not breathing normally** is in cardiac arrest and requires CPR.

Immediately following cardiac arrest blood flow to the brain is reduced to virtually zero, which may cause seizure-like episodes that may be confused with epilepsy.

You should be suspicious of cardiac arrest with any casualty that presents seizure like symptoms and carefully assess whether they are breathing normally.

PAGE 34 | SECTION 16

BONES, JOINTS AND MUSCLE INJURIES

FIRST AID AT WORK

The human skeleton is made up of 206 bones, the largest being the femur, or thigh bone.

It serves many purposes:
- It protects vital organs such as the brain, heart and lungs
- It supports muscles held to the skeleton by tendons
- It provides movement in the form of joints which are held together by ligaments

There are three types of joints:
1. Non-movable - such as the bones that make up the skull
2. Partially movable - such as the ribs and spine
3. Movable joints - such as the hip, which is made up of a ball and socket

Through various activities, bones can be damaged or broken.

Breaks or fractures fall into three main categories:
1. Closed fracture. This is where the break does not penetrate the skin
2. Open fracture. This is where the broken bone does penetrate the skin
3. Complicated fracture. This is where the broken bone injures another part of the body i.e. a broken rib penetrating a lung

In respect of first aid, there is nothing you can do to repair the fracture. However, you can offer treatment that will make the casualty more comfortable in order to prevent the injury from worsening.

DO NOT attempt to straighten or realign a fracture.

Your aims are to:
- Prevent movement of the broken bone
- Support them in the position found
- Call 999 for the emergency services
- Limit their pain
- Reduce the chance of further injury
- Facilitate safe and prompt transport

Skull

The Skeleton
Supports the muscles, blood vessels and nerves of the body, as well as protecting the organs

The Muscles
Allows various parts of the body to move

Ligaments
Hold moveable joints together

The Joints
Where one bone meets the other

Tendons
Hold muscle to the bone

CLOSED FRACTURE

Signs and symptoms
- Pain
- Swelling
- Deformity
- Internal bleeding
- Bruising
- Shock

Treatment
- Immobilise the injured part to stop any movement
- Place padding around the injury for further support
- Leave the casualty in the position found unless they can move the injured part to a more comfortable position
- For additional support, particularly if there is a delay in the emergency services arriving, you could consider strapping an uninjured leg to the injured one. Use broad-fold bandages and ensure that any knots are tied to the uninjured side. Do not wrap a bandage over the fracture. If their circulation is impaired, loosen the dressings
- You MUST NOT try to realign the fracture. This should only be performed by medically trained professionals
- Do not give you casualty anything to eat or drink
- Treat for shock
- Call 999/112

SECTION 17 | PAGE 35

BONES, JOINTS AND MUSCLE INJURIES continued

SUPPORT SLING

Fractures to the lower arm and wrist are a common injury. In adults, it accounts for approximately half of all broken bones. In children, fractures of the forearm are second only to broken collarbones.

There is little a First Aider can do other than support it and to dispatch them to hospital.

In respect of support, generally speaking the casualty will support it themselves, and will not want you to move it.

If they are unable to support it themselves, then you can offer to apply a support sling using a triangular bandage.

Identify the injury to the arm and providing the arm can be bent at the elbow, offer your casualty a support for it.

Pass the bandage under the injured arm with the long base running parallel with the body. The point opposite the long base should be at the elbow of the injured arm.

Bring the lower point of the bandage up over the injured arm and over the shoulder so that the two ends meet.

Tie off the two ends on the injured side above the collar bone. Place the two ends under the knot to act as a cushion for the knot.

Secure the trailing bandage at the elbow with a safety pin, or by twisting it fairly tight and losing it by tucking it away within the sling.

Ensure that there is still circulation in the fingertips by performing a capillary refill check. Press a fingernail which should go pale. When released it should go back to normal colouration. Transport them to the hospital or call 999 if they are unable to walk.

ELEVATED SLING FOR FOREARM AND HAND INJURIES

OPEN FRACTURE

Signs and symptoms
- Pain
- Deformity
- Internal bleeding
- External bleeding
- Shock

Treatment
- Call for an ambulance immediately
- Prevent any movement
- Reduce the risk of infection by wearing gloves
- Control the blood loss by dressing around the wound
- DO NOT apply any direct pressure on the protruding bone
- Use sterile non-fluffy dressings
- For additional support, particularly if there is a delay in the emergency services arriving, you could consider strapping an uninjured leg to the injured one.

  Use broad-fold bandages and ensure that any knots are tied to the uninjured side. Do not wrap a bandage over the fracture. If their circulation is impaired, loosen the dressings
- You MUST NOT try to realign the fracture. This should only be performed by medically trained professionals
- Treat for shock
- Monitor their vital signs
- Do not offer the casualty anything to eat, drink or smoke as a general anaesthetic may have to be administered when they get to hospital

COMPLICATED FRACTURE

Signs and symptoms
- Pain
- Deformity
- Internal and external bleeding
- Shock

Treatment
- Call for an ambulance immediately
- Apply the same treatment as mentioned before for an open or closed fracture
- Be aware of a possible secondary injury which may not be visible. An example of this could be a fractured rib which may have affected an internal organ
- Monitor them very closely and be prepared to resuscitate them

DISLOCATIONS

Dislocations are extremely painful and are often caused by a violent muscle contraction, a strong force wrenching the bone into an abnormal position, or even as something as simple as turning over in bed can cause it.

The recognition of a dislocation is that of a fracture, with the addition of disfigurement around the joint.

In all cases, the ligaments holding the bones together will be damaged.

Under no circumstances should you try to put the dislocated joint back into place.

You must send your casualty to hospital for treatment.

Signs and symptoms
- Severe pain
- Swelling and bruising around the affected joint
- Difficulty in moving the affected area
- The affected area may look twisted or shortened

Treatment

If the casualty does not want the limb strapped or supported with a sling, then allow them to support it themselves, if this is possible, and transport them to hospital.

BONES, JOINTS AND MUSCLE INJURIES continued

SPRAINS AND STRAINS

These are most commonly associated with sports injuries, or when a person moves suddenly and exerts a great deal of pressure on the muscles or joints. It's sometimes difficult to distinguish between the type of soft tissue injury and a fracture, because of the pain and swelling. If you are unsure, you should suspect the worse and treat for a fracture.

Sprains and strains are collectively known as soft tissue injuries.

SPRAIN

A sprain occurs when one or more of the ligaments have been stretched, twisted, or torn, usually as a result of excessive force being applied to a joint.

The most common locations for a sprain to occur are:

- **The knee** - which can become strained when a person turns quickly during sports or other physical activities
- **The ankle** - which can become strained when walking or running on an uneven surface
- **The wrist** - which can become strained when a person falls onto their hand
- **The thumb** - which can become strained during intense and repetitive physical activity, such as playing a racquet sport

STRAIN

A strain occurs when the muscle fibres stretch or tear. They usually occur for one of two reasons:

- **When the muscle has been stretched beyond its limits**
- **When the muscle has been forced to contract** (shorten too quickly)

Strains can develop as the result of an accident, or during physical or sporting activities, such as running or playing football.

Signs and symptoms for both sprains and strains
- Pain
- Swelling
- Bruising
- Inflammation
- **Cramp** (Strains)

Treatment

Firstly, protect the injury from worsening. Asking the casualty to walk or run off the injury could seriously jeopardise the extent of the injury!

PROTECT the injured area from further injury by using a support or (in the case of an ankle injury) wearing shoes that enclose and support the feet, such as lace-ups.

REST by stopping the activity that caused the injury and rest the injured joint or muscle. Avoid activity for the first 48 to 72 hours after the injury was afflicted.

ICE - for the first 48 to 72 hours after the injury, apply ice wrapped in a damp towel to the injured area for 15 to 20 minutes every two to three hours during the day. Do not leave the ice on whilst sleeping, and do not allow the ice to touch the skin directly, because it could cause a cold burn.

COMPRESS or bandage the injured area to limit any swelling and movement that could damage it further. Use a simple elastic bandage or elasticated tubular bandage. It should be wrapped snuggly around the affected area, but not so tightly that it restricts blood flow. Remove the bandage before going to sleep.

ELEVATION - keep the injured area raised and supported to help reduce swelling.

The most common types of strains are:

- **Hamstring strains** - the hamstrings are muscles that run down the back of the leg and are connected to the hip and knee joints
- **Calf muscle strains** - the gastrocnemius and soleus are the medical names for the muscles of the calf located between the ankle and the knee at the back of the leg
- **Quadriceps strains** - the quadriceps are muscles located at the front of the thigh
- **Lumbar strains** - the lumbar muscles are found in the lower back

HEAD AND SPINAL INJURIES

If someone is unable to respond to people or activities, then they are deemed as being unresponsive.

Unresponsiveness can be caused by any major illness or injury as well as substance abuse and alcohol use. These conditions include head injuries, poisoning, hypothermia, heatstroke, epilepsy, diabetes, heart attack, stroke and shock. This is by no means the definitive list and this section addresses just some of these conditions.

All injuries to the head are potentially dangerous and they all require a medical assessment.

During any assessment of a head injury, or unresponsiveness, it is useful to record and monitor the casualty by using an observation chart (see page 14).

You should be monitoring and looking at the following:

- Eyes
- Speech
- Movement
- Breathing
- Responsiveness

Your objective throughout this monitoring process, is to note any changes in the condition of your casualty in respect of improvement or deterioration.

Although this scale is designed for checks to be made every ten minutes, you should carry out constant monitoring of a casualty until the emergency services take over from you.

CONCUSSION

A concussion is a traumatic brain injury that may result in a bad headache, altered levels of alertness, or unresponsiveness.

It temporarily interferes with the way your brain works, and it can affect memory, judgment, reflexes, speech, balance, coordination, and sleep patterns.

Signs and symptoms

The most common signs and symptoms of concussion are:

- **Evidence of a head injury** (blood or bruising)
- **Headache and nausea**
- **Dizziness and loss of balance**
- **Confusion, such as being unaware of your surroundings**
- **Feeling stunned or dazed**
- **Disturbances with vision, such as double vision or seeing "stars" or flashing lights**
- **Difficulties with memory**

Treatment

- If they are responsive, rest them by sitting them down, or lying them down with their head raised and hold a cold compress against the injury
- Keep them warm and keep talking to them
- Ensure the cold compress stays on the injury for no longer than 20 minutes
- Monitor their airway, breathing and response levels
- If they are unresponsive, you must call for an ambulance and support them in the position found
- You must recommend that they seek medical advice, particularly if they develop a headache, feel sick or they sleep more than they would normally do

CEREBRAL COMPRESSION

This very serious condition is due to pressure being exerted on the brain from a build-up of blood or fluid, blood clot, or depressed as a result of a skull fracture.

This may follow on from concussion either directly, or at some point after their apparent recovery. For this reason, all head injuries must be examined by medical personnel.

Signs and symptoms

- **Their response levels will deteriorate, possibly leading to unresponsiveness**
- **Signs of a recent head injury**
- **Severe headache**
  - **Weakness and/or paralysis down one side of the face or body**
    - **Flushed face and high temperature**
    - **Drowsiness**
    - **Behavioural changes**
    - **Slow noisy breathing**
- **Unequal pupil sizes**

Treatment

- Call for an ambulance immediately
- If they are responsive, keep them supported in a comfortable position by lying them down with their head and shoulders raised, providing injuries allow, and keeping them warm
- Monitor their response levels
- If they become unresponsive, check their breathing and carry out your basic life support procedures dependant on the result

HEAD AND SPINAL INJURIES continued

SKULL FRACTURE

A skull fracture can be caused by a heavy blow to the head, which may result in a depressed fracture of the skull, or by landing awkwardly from a fall or collision resulting in a base skull fracture. There may also be a wound allowing infection inside the skull. There may also be evidence of concussion and compression.

Signs and symptoms
- Evidence of trauma to the head
- Possible depression of the skull
- Bruising around the head
- Clear fluid or watery blood coming from the nose or ear
- Bloodshot eyes
- Deterioration of response levels

Treatment
- If you suspect a spinal injury, do not move them
- Lay them down, head and shoulders raised if you are able to move them, injured side down
- Call for an ambulance
- Monitor their airway, breathing and response levels
- Cover their ear with a sterile dressing if there is fluid running out of it
- Control the bleeding and fluid loss
- All head injuries must be advised to go to hospital

SPINAL INJURIES

The spine, also known as the backbone, is a strong, flexible column of ring-like bones that runs from our skull to our pelvis. It holds the head and body upright and allows us to bend and twist our body. It also offers protection to our spinal cord - a large bundle of nerves that runs through the cavity in the centre of our spine that relays messages between our brain and the rest of our body.

It is made up of 33 irregularly shaped bones called vertebrae.

Each vertebra has a hole in the middle through which the spinal cord runs.

The spine can be divided into five different regions, from top to bottom:

1. Seven cervical vertebrae support our head and neck and allow us to nod and shake our head
2. Our ribs are attached to our 12 thoracic vertebrae
3. Our five sturdy lumbar vertebrae carry most of the weight of our upper body and provide a stable centre of gravity when we move
4. Our sacrum is made up of five fused vertebrae. It makes up the back wall of our pelvis
5. Our coccyx is made up of four fused vertebrae. It is an evolutionary remnant of the tail found in most other vertebrates

Shock absorbers

Sandwiched between our vertebrae are pads of tough, fibrous cartilage called inter-vertebral discs that cushion our vertebrae and absorb shock. These discs, together with the curved 'S' shape of our spine, prevents shock to our head when we walk or run.

Any damage to our spine can not only be life-threatening, but it can also leave us permanently damaged. It can lead to paralysis to parts of our body that is irreparable.

Therefore, your handling of your casualty where you suspect a spinal injury is critical in ensuring that their condition does not worsen.

Spinal discs, 23 in total are located between the vertebrae

- 7 Cervical vertebrae
- 12 Thoracic vertebrae
- 5 Lumbar vertebrae
- Coccyx

FIRST AID AT WORK

Signs and symptoms

When the spinal column or vertebrae are damaged:

- An unusual curvature of the spine
- Pain at the site of injury. Be aware that this may be masked by other pains in other parts of the body
- Tenderness in the skin that covers the spine

When the spinal cord is damaged:

- No control over limb movement
- Loss of sensation, or abnormal sensations such as numbness, burning or tingling
- The casualty may say that the limbs feel heavy or clumsy
- Loss of bladder and bowel control
- Breathing difficulties

Treatment

- Call for an ambulance immediately
- Prevent any movement and support in the position found
- Support their head throughout but do not cover the ears with your hands, as this will impair their hearing
- Monitor their breathing and other vital signs whilst you are waiting for the ambulance to arrive
- Be prepared to resuscitate

SECTION 18 | PAGE 41

CHEST AND ABDOMINAL INJURIES

PENETRATING CHEST WOUNDS

Contained within the chest cavity is the heart and the lungs. These extremely important organs are protected by a ribcage made up of 12 pairs of ribs and the breastbone (sternum).
In addition, the ribcage is of sufficient size to give protection to other vital organs such as the liver and spleen.

Any wound to the chest could therefore, cause life-threatening damage. These include, penetrating wounds such as a stabbing or a broken rib. An injury that you may not necessarily see could also inflict major damage to any of these organs, and therefore your prompt and effective treatment is vital in preserving life and in preventing the injury from worsening.

Signs and symptoms
- Obvious signs of trauma – blood loss
- Shortness of breath
- Respiratory distress
- Chest pain
- Shock
- **Cyanosis** (blueness around the extremities such as the ears and lips)
- Swelling
- Chest wall bruising
- Open wounds
- Distended neck veins
- **Tracheal deviation** (shifting of the windpipe)

In addition, you may see evidence of the following:
- 'Bubbling' around the wound
- Coughed up red frothy blood
- The sound of air being sucked in when the casualty breathes

Treatment
- Wear medical gloves
- Help the casualty to sit down on the floor and lean them towards the injured side.
- Do not cover the wound. Leave it exposed. However, if the wound is bleeding, you must apply direct pressure to the wound and apply a non-occlusive dressing if it is necessary
- If there is something embedded, build up padding on either side of the object until it is high enough for you to be able to bandage over the top of the object without pressing it further into the wound. If you cannot build padding high enough, build around the object with rolled sterile dressings and secure in place to control the loss of blood
- Treat for shock by sitting them on the floor, supported and leaning towards the injured side
- Ring for an ambulance immediately

RIBCAGE INJURY

The ribcage can be damaged by a crush, a direct blow to the chest or by falling.

It has been known for a rib to be broken by coughing excessively!

Flail chest is a life-threatening medical condition that occurs when a segment of the rib cage breaks due to trauma and becomes detached from the rest of the chest wall. Two of the symptoms of flail chest are chest pain and shortness of breath.

It is an extremely painful injury, but the concerns are for the vital organs that are contained within the ribcage. Because of this, you may well have to deal with a potentially life-threatening injury such as a punctured lung or internal bleeding.

Treatment

- Sit the casualty down and support them
- Lean them towards the injured side, but comfortably in a position that suits them
- If the casualty allows, apply an elevated sling to the arm on the injured side. Do not enforce this if the injury is so painful that they would prefer to support it themselves
- Call for an ambulance
- If the casualty becomes unresponsive, support them in the position found unless you believe their airway is at risk, then you should place them in the recovery position injured side down, taking extreme care when rolling them over
- Monitor their airway and breathing

CRUSH INJURY

These are most common on construction sites or in road traffic accidents.

However, natural disasters such as earthquakes and tsunamis will also have its casualties. In war torn areas, collapsed buildings and upturned vehicles will also increase the risk of numerous casualties that are crushed.

Treatment for casualties that have been crushed for LESS THAN 15 MINUTES

- If it's possible, release the casualty from the crush as soon as you can
- Remember your first aid priorities and treat appropriately
- Breathing
- Bleeding
- Burns and breaks
- Treat for shock
- Call 999/112 for an ambulance

Treatment for casualties that have been crushed for MORE THAN 15 MINUTES

- Do not remove the item that is crushing your casualty
- Call for an ambulance
- Monitor the casualty's breathing and response levels
- Offer them plenty of reassurance
- Treat them for shock

**The reason for not releasing the casualty after 15 minutes of being crushed is that toxins will build around the muscle area that is crushed.
These potentially life-threatening toxins will be released into the blood stream that could prove to be fatal.**

CHEST AND ABDOMINAL INJURIES continued

ABDOMINAL INJURIES
Abdominal wounds

If your casualty has been injured by a stabbing, a gunshot or by any other cause that would create a penetrating wound, then your priority is to ensure that the casualty is breathing normally and then to control the blood loss.

If there is anything penetrating from the wound such as a knife, then it must be left in place and the wound dressed around it using sterile dressings.

It is important to wear gloves as in any type of incident involving blood loss.

Signs and symptoms
- Evidence of blood loss
- Pain
- Possible entry and exit wound with a high velocity wound such as a gun shot
- Shock
- Possible embedded object
- Possible shortness of breath

Treatment
- If the casualty is responsive, then lie them down with their knees raised and supported
- Loosen tight clothing
- Dress the wound/s with a sterile dressing and secure it with adhesive tape
- Call for an ambulance
- If blood seeps through the first dressing, then remove it and apply a new one and secure it in place
- Treat for shock and monitor their breathing and responsiveness
- If the casualty becomes unresponsive, support them in the position found unless you believe their airway is at risk, then you should place them in the recovery position injured side down

In extreme cases, it is important to ensure that the contents of the abdomen are contained within the abdominal cavity, particularly if the casualty vomits or coughs. Hold a sterile dressing firmly in place over the wound to prevent the contents from spilling out. Be prepared to resuscitate, should they stop breathing normally.

Abdominal pains

Abdominal pains can be brought on by many reasons. In less serious cases, such as stomach ache, then the casualty will normally recover without the intervention of medical assistance. Most will recover quickly by lying down with the comfort of a hot water bottle on their tummy.

If the pain is severe, and it induces vomiting or diarrhoea, then you should contact a doctor.

If the pain is so severe that it causes the casualty to 'double up' in pain, particularly if the pain comes in 'waves', then you should summon an ambulance immediately.

SPECIALISED BURN INJURIES

Treating chemical burns

If your casualty is suffering a burn from a chemical, a bleach or acid you should:

- If the burn is severe, dial 999 immediately for urgent help
- Wear protective gloves to prevent contact with the chemical
- Flush the affected area continuously (for at least 20 minutes) with as much clean water as possible
- Try to make sure the water can run off the affected area without pooling on the skin
- If the chemical is dry, brush it off the skin
- Remove any jewellery or clothing that may have been exposed to the chemical
- Stay on the phone until the ambulance arrives and follow any other advice given by the 999 call handler to avoid further injury
- If the burn is minor, take your casualty to hospital for the extent of the burn to be assessed

ELECTRICITY

Electrical burns can be caused by lightning or from a man made source involving either, a high-voltage supply e.g. overhead power lines, or from a low-voltage supply as found in the home, or at work.

In all cases, an electrical injury can be life-threatening.

You may have multiple injuries to treat, including cessation of breathing, and a wound that enters the body as well as one that exits the body.

Your first priority is to ensure that it is safe to offer your casualty treatment.

In respect of a high-voltage injury, it is imperative that you and all bystanders stay well away from your casualty. Because the supply can 'arc', you must stay at least 18 metres away from the supply source.

You must call the emergency services immediately, detailing the extent of the incident.

In some cases of low-voltage injuries, the casualty may still have a contact with the supply, and therefore be 'live'. You must break the source of supply immediately before attempting any form of treatment. Switch the supply off from the main fuse-board. Failing that, remove the electrical device from the casualty. You can achieve this by standing on a dry insulating material such as a book or telephone directory. Use a wooden or plastic handle to drag away the source from the casualty ensuring that the area is safe for all.

As soon as you have deemed it safe to do so, you may start your treatment.

Treatment
LIGHTNING STRIKE

Only when it is safe to do so:

- Carry out your basic life support procedures
- Call for the emergency services
- Be aware of any potential serious burns to deal with

HIGH-VOLTAGE INJURIES

- Keep everyone at least 18 metres away from the electrical source
- Call for the emergency services
- Only when it is safe to do so, as directed by the emergency services, carry out your basic life support procedures

LOW-VOLTAGE INJURIES

- Switch off from the MAINS supply
- Break contact between the electricity and your casualty
- If you are unable to do this, you must insulate yourself before attempting to free your casualty from the supply

Once your casualty is free from the supply:

- Carry out your basic life support procedures
- Call for the emergency services
- Be aware of any potential serious burns to deal with

EYE INJURIES

EYE INJURIES

Eye injuries have a number of different causes, such as a blow to the eye, foreign bodies, lacerations (cuts) and ultraviolet light.

Eye injuries can also be caused by chemical exposures and burns as a result of liquid being splashed into the eyes.

Some aerosols can be harmful to the eyes, including Mace (attack defence spray), tear gas, pepper spray and some chemicals in hair spray. Chemicals can also be transferred from the skin on your hands to your eyes.

A BLOW TO THE EYE

Serious and permanent eye damage can result from a blunt object, from a sports injury, a fall or a fight. Care should be taken when treating such an injury as the bone surrounding the eye could be fractured.

Signs and symptoms
- Pain
- Swelling
- Bruising
- Possible bleeding
- Redness of the eye
- Headache

Treatment
When to seek medical help.

Send your casualty to see their GP if:
- They have a change in vision
- The pain is persistent
- There is pus or warmth and redness, indicating infection
- They become forgetful or drowsy
- They have nausea, vomiting and/or dizziness
- The swelling does not subside after a few days

Go to your hospital accident and emergency department if:
- They have two black eyes (this could suggest a skull fracture)
- They have double vision
- They cannot move the eye
- They think something has pierced the eye
- There is a cut to the eye or blood inside the eye
- Fluid is leaking from the eye or the eye looks deformed
- They are taking blood-thinning medication such as aspirin, or have a bleeding disorder such as haemophilia

FOREIGN BODIES IN THE EYE

Foreign bodies, such as metal, plastic or wood, can scratch or graze the surface of the eye or cornea.

Examples of foreign bodies that can cause a corneal abrasion include being poked in the eye by a finger or hot cigarette ash flying into the eye.

In severe cases, the foreign body may be embedded.

Signs and symptoms
- Sensation that something is in the eye
- Increase in tears produced by the eye
- Pain
- Blurred or double vision
- Sensitivity to light
- A visible foreign body on the cornea
- A rust ring or stain on the cornea if the foreign body is metal

Treatment
- Sit the casualty down, and stand behind them
- Lean their head back and very gently separate their eyelid with your finger and thumb and inspect the eye
- If you can see the foreign object, then try flushing it out with a sterile eye wash solution, or clean tap water. Place a towel on the shoulder on the side of the injured eye. Lean the head back and inclined towards the injured side. Gently pour the eye wash into the eye to flush it out
- If this doesn't work, then you must seek medical advice

Embedded Objects in the Eye

If there is something embedded, then you must leave it in place. Cover the eye with a sterile dressing, being extremely careful not to make any contact with the foreign body that is embedded. Transport them to hospital immediately, or ring for an ambulance.

FIRST AID AT WORK

LACERATIONS OF THE EYE

Eye lacerations can be caused by falls, contact with sharp objects, particularly flying objects such as grit, debris from a garden strimmer and shards of glass.

Signs and symptoms
- Eye pain and sensitivity to light
- Increase in tears produced by the eye
- Blurred or distorted vision
- Squinting caused by spasm of the muscle surrounding the eye
- Feeling that something is in the eye and it cannot be removed

Treatment
- Lie the casualty down and support their head in order to rest them. Try to keep both their eyes still
- Cover their injured eye with a sterile eye dressing, or ask them to hold a sterile dressing in place
- Take them to the hospital if you are able to transport them. Failing that, call for an ambulance immediately

ULTRAVIOLET LIGHT

Ultraviolet (UV) light can lead to an eye injury called corneal flash burn. Exposure to the sun, glare from a welder's torch and sun lamps can cause of this type of injury. It could also affect both eyes.

Signs and symptoms
- Pain
- Redness and watering
- A gritty feeling
- Sensitive to light

Treatment
- Cover the eye with a sterile eye dressing
- Take them to the hospital if you are able to transport them. Failing that, call for an ambulance immediately

CHEMICAL BURNS TO THE EYES

The surface of the eye can be severely damaged with any type of chemical burn. It can lead to the loss of sight if it is not treated quickly.

Chemicals can be transferred to the eye by splashing, spraying or simply from your own finger should it be contaminated.

Signs and symptoms
- Watering of the eye
- Pain
- Swelling
- Redness
- Evidence of the chemical

Treatment
- You must wear gloves to prevent yourself being contaminated by the chemical
- Irrigate the eye for at least 20 minutes under running cool water, either by holding the head under a running tap, or by flushing the eye with a continual supply of cool tap water from a suitable container
- Ensure that the irrigation does not flow into the other eye
- Try to identify the chemical so that the emergency services know what chemical they are treating
- Cover the injured eye with a sterile eye dressing
- Arrange to transport them to hospital, or call for an ambulance

POISONING

Poisoning happens when you take into your body, a substance that damages your cells and organs, and injures your health.

Poisons are usually swallowed, but they can also be absorbed through the skin, injected, inhaled or splashed into the eyes.

Many substances are only poisonous if an abnormally large amount is taken. For example, paracetamol is harmless if you take one or two tablets for a headache, but is poisonous if you take an overdose.

A poison can enter the body in a number of ways:
- **Swallowed**   Food, alcohol, drugs etc.
- **Absorbed**   Chemicals, vapours etc. through the skin
- **Injected**   Drugs, medicine, stings etc.
- **Inhaled**   Gases, fumes etc
- **Splashed**   into the eyes. Chemicals, etc.

General treatment for poisons
- Call for an ambulance immediately
- Place in the recovery position in order to maintain an open airway, and to allow vomit to drain from the mouth
- Keep any evidence of the poison
- Monitor their breathing and be prepared to resuscitate them

HOUSEHOLD POISONS

Bleach, oven cleaner, paint stripper etc

Recognition if it is swallowed
- **Redness, blistering, burns and swelling to the face, mouth and lips**
- **Distressed breathing, leading to unresponsiveness**

Treatment
- **Check the airway and their breathing. Be prepared to resuscitate** (use a face shield)
- **Call for an ambulance**
- If they are unresponsive, place them in the recovery position and monitor their breathing while waiting for the ambulance to arrive
- Identify the poison that was taken
- Do not induce vomiting

INDUSTRIAL POISONS

Corrosive chemicals and gases

Recognition
- Possible burning sensation in the airway and skin
- Breathing difficulties
- Burns around the body
- Possible coughing and sneezing
- Nausea and vomiting
- Severe headache and disorientation
- Unresponsiveness

Treatment
- Call for an ambulance immediately
- Protect yourself
- Remove the casualty from the source
- Move them into fresh air
- Treat the appropriate condition such as a burn
- If they become unresponsive, place them in the recovery position and monitor their breathing
- Be prepared to resuscitate them

DRUG POISONING OR OVERDOSE

Recognition

ASPIRIN
- Upper abdominal pain
- Nausea and vomiting
- Ringing in the ears
- Confusion and delirium
- 'Sighing' when breathing
- Dizziness

PARACETAMOL
- Developing abdominal pains
- Nausea and vomiting

TRANQUILLISERS
- Lethargy, sleepiness leading to unresponsiveness
- Shallow breathing
- Weak, irregular pulse

NARCOTICS
- Small pupils
- Sluggishness and confusion, possibly leading to unresponsiveness
- Slow, shallow breathing which may stop
- Needle marks which may be infected

SOLVENTS
- Nausea and vomiting
- Headaches
- Hallucinations
- Unresponsiveness – possibly

STIMULANTS
- Excitable, hyperactive behaviour, wildness and frenzy
- Sweating
- Tremors
- Hallucinations

Treatment
- Protect yourself
- If responsive, place them in a comfortable position and try to establish the drug that has been taken
- Call for an ambulance
- Monitor their breathing
- Keep samples of vomited material and try to find evidence of the drug that was taken
- Be prepared to resuscitate

POISONING continued

PLANT POISONING

Most plants that grow in the UK are harmless and, if eaten, may only cause a mild stomach upset.

Some types of plant can have a more serious effect, so it is important to know what plants are growing in your garden.

If a potentially poisonous plant has been eaten, try to identify it so you can inform medical staff, or take a sample with you to the hospital so that it can be identified.

The plants to look out for include, Wild Arum, Foxglove, Laburnum, Death Cap mushrooms, Ivy and Mistletoe - to name a few.

Recognition
- Nausea and vomiting
- Abdominal pains
- Diarrhoea
- Seizures
- Impaired responsiveness

Treatment

The same treatment can be applied as you would for drug poisoning (see page 49).

FOOD POISONING

This is usually caused by consuming contaminated food or drink. Some food poisoning is caused by foods that already have the bacteria in it, particularly from the E.Coli or salmonella group of bacteria.

This particular poison could take hours or days before it takes effect.

The other main group are poisons produced by staphylococcus. The symptoms of poisoning develop far more rapidly, normally within 2-6 hours.

Recognition
- Nausea and vomiting
- Abdominal pains
- Diarrhoea
- Fever
- Headache
- Impaired responsiveness

Treatment
- Encourage the casualty to rest
- Offer them plenty of bland fluids to drink
- Try to establish the source of the poisoning in case medical assistance is required
- Call for an ambulance if their condition deteriorates

ALCOHOL POISONING

Alcohol poisoning results from drinking a toxic amount of alcohol, usually over a short period of time, which is known as binge drinking.

On rare occasions, alcohol poisoning can occur if you accidentally drink household products that contain alcohol.

The intake of alcohol depresses the activity of the central nervous system, particularly the brain. Prolonged or excessive intake can severely impair all physical and mental functions and the casualty may become unresponsive.

Recognition
- Smell of alcohol
- Evidence of empty containers
- Impaired unresponsiveness, leading to unresponsiveness
- Flushed appearance
- Deep, noisy breathing

In the later stages of unresponsiveness:
- Dry, bloated appearance to the face
- Shallow breathing
- Weak and rapid pulse
- Dilated pupils

Treatment
- Place them in the recovery position to maintain an open airway
- Monitor their breathing
- Keep them warm
- Seek medical assistance if there is another condition, such as a head injury to deal with

NATIONAL POISONS INFORMATION SERVICE (NPIS)

In an emergency, members of the public should always contact their general practitioners, NHS 24, NHS Direct or local A&E department. If your casualty has collapsed, or is not breathing properly, you must call for an ambulance immediately, by dialling 999, and then carry out your basic life support treatment.

The NPIS does not provide poisons information directly to members of the public. Therefore, for routine poisons advice you should contact your general practitioner or telephone NHS Direct on 111.

Should you require specific information on poisons in the Republic of Ireland, contact the National Poisons Information Centre on 01 809 2166.

The Control of Substances Hazardous to Health (COSHH) Regulations.

Many materials or substances used or created at work could harm your health. These substances could be dusts, gases or fumes that you breathe in, or liquids, gels or powders that come into contact with your eyes or skin. There could also be harmful micro-organisms (more commonly known as germs) present that can cause infection, an allergic reaction or are toxic.

Harmful substances can be present in anything from paints and cleaners to flour dust, solder fume, blood or waste. Ill health caused by these substances used at work is preventable.

Many substances can harm health but, used properly, they almost never do.

The law requires you to adequately control exposure to materials in the workplace that cause ill health. This means:

- Identifying which harmful substances may be present in the workplace
- Deciding how workers might be exposed to them and be harmed
- Looking at what measures you have in place to prevent this harm and deciding whether you are doing enough
- Providing information, instruction and training
- In appropriate cases, providing health surveillance

ANAPHYLAXIS

Any allergic reaction including the most extreme form, anaphylactic shock, occurs because the body's immune system reacts inappropriately in response to the presence of a substance that it wrongly perceives as a threat.

An anaphylactic reaction is caused by the sudden release of chemical substances, including histamine, from cells in the blood and tissues where they are stored. The release is triggered by the reaction between the allergic antibody (IgE) and the substance (allergen) causing the anaphylactic reaction. This mechanism is so sensitive that minute quantities of the allergen can cause a reaction. The released chemicals react on blood vessels to cause the swelling in the mouth and anywhere on the skin. There is a fall in blood pressure and, in asthmatics; the effect is mainly on the lungs.

WHAT CAN CAUSE ANAPHYLAXIS?

Common causes include foods such as peanuts, tree nuts (e.g. almonds, walnuts, cashews, Brazils), sesame, fish, shellfish, dairy products and eggs. Non-food causes include wasp or bee stings, natural latex (rubber), penicillin or any other drug or injection. For some people, exercise can trigger a severe reaction - either on its own or in combination with other factors such as food or drugs (e.g. aspirin).

Signs and symptoms

The symptoms of anaphylaxis usually start between 3 and 60 minutes after contact with the allergen. Less commonly, they can occur a few hours or even days after contact.

When your casualty has an anaphylactic reaction, they may feel unwell or dizzy or may faint because of a sudden drop in blood pressure.

Narrowing of the airways can also occur at the same time, with or without the drop in blood pressure. This can cause breathing difficulties and wheezing.

Your casualty may also experience any of the symptoms below:

- **Swollen eyes, lips, hands, feet and other areas**
- **A strange metallic taste in the mouth**
- **Sore, red, itchy eyes**
- **Changes in heart rate**
- **A sudden feeling of extreme anxiety or apprehension**
- **Itchy skin or nettle-rash** (hives)
- **Unresponsiveness due to very low blood pressure**
- **Abdominal cramps, vomiting or diarrhoea**
- **Nausea and fever**

Your casualty would not necessarily experience all of these symptoms.

Adrenaline is the gold standard in the treatment of anaphylaxis, and its administration should not be delayed.

In a first aid situation, adrenalin will normally be delivered by an auto-injector.

If available, an injection of adrenaline should be given as soon as possible.

If after 5 minutes the casualty still feels unwell, a second injection should be given. This should be given in the opposite thigh.

A second dose may also be required if the symptoms reoccur.

When treating a potential anaphylaxis casualty, it should be noted that there are **NO** contraindications for the use of adrenaline.

Treatment for a severe reaction

- **Use an adrenaline auto-injector if the person has one**
- **Call 999 for an ambulance immediately (even if they start to feel better) – mention that you think the person has anaphylaxis**
- **Lie the person down flat – unless they are unresponsive, pregnant or having breathing difficulties**
- **Give another injection after 5 minutes if the symptoms do not improve and a second auto-injector is available. This should be given in the opposite thigh**
- **If they become unresponsive, place them in the recovery position and be prepared to resuscitate them if they stop breathing normally**

What the HSE say:

Some workers carry their own medication that has been prescribed by their doctor (e.g. an inhaler for asthma). If an individual needs to take their own prescribed medication, the First Aider's role is generally limited to helping them to do so and contacting the emergency services as appropriate.

However, this does not apply to the administration of prescription only medication specified in Schedule 19 of the Medicines Regulations 2012, where this is for the purpose of saving life in an emergency. Adrenaline 1:1000 up to 1 mg for intramuscular use in anaphylaxis is an example.

Where a first aid needs assessment identifies that Schedule 19 medication may be required to be administered in an emergency, the employer should consider providing workplace First Aiders with additional training in their use.

MAJOR ILLNESSES

HEART ATTACK

A heart attack is a serious medical condition in which the supply of blood to the heart is suddenly blocked, usually by a blood clot. The lack of blood to the heart can seriously damage the heart muscles. If left untreated, the muscles will begin to die. The medical term for a heart attack is myocardial infarction.

Most heart attacks occur in people with coronary heart disease, which is caused by a serious condition where the arteries become narrowed and hardened by the build-up of clumps of cholesterol, called plaques.

The two arteries that supply the heart are called the coronary arteries. People with hardened and narrowed coronary arteries are said to have coronary heart disease (CHD).

Risk factors for CHD include:
- Smoking
- High-fat diet
- Diabetes
- Being overweight or obesity

Heart attacks are very common and are one of the leading causes of death in England. Each year in England, an estimated 111,000 people have a heart attack. Many heart attacks that lead to death are preventable. This is because most of the risk factors that are listed above can also be prevented.

Most heart attacks occur in people who are over 45 years of age. Men are two to three times more likely to have a heart attack than women.

Signs and symptoms

The symptoms of a heart attack can include:
- Pale blue/grey, cold and clammy skin
- Chest pain. The pain is usually located in the centre of the chest and can feel like a sensation of pressure, tightness or squeezing
- Pain in other parts of the body. It can feel as if the pain is travelling from the chest to the arms (usually the left arm is affected, but it can affect both arms), jaw, neck, back and abdomen
- Shortness of breath
- Nausea
- An overwhelming sense of anxiety (similar to having a panic attack)
- Feeling light headed
- Coughing
- Vomiting
- Wheezing

Treatment
- Make the casualty comfortable and warm
- Position them in the half-sitting position
- Monitor their breathing
- Call for an ambulance
- Calm and reassure them
- If they become unresponsive, you must open their airway and check for normal breathing, and be prepared to resuscitate them

ANGINA

Angina is a heart condition that is caused when the blood supply to the muscles of the heart is restricted. It usually occurs when the arteries that supply the heart become hardened and narrowed.

The main symptom of angina is a dull, heavy or tight pain in the chest that can sometimes spread to the left arm, neck, jaw or back. The pain is usually triggered by physical activity or stress and usually only lasts for a few minutes.

The onset of this type of chest pain is often referred to as an angina attack.

The signs and symptoms are very similar to that of a heart attack, and if you are unsure about their condition, you should offer them treatment as you would for a heart attack victim.

Treating angina

There are three main goals in treating angina.

They are:
- **To relieve the symptoms during an angina attack by resting and re-assuring them**
- **To help them administer their own medication if they have it**
- **To call 999/112 for medical assistance if there is no improvement**

> You can assist your casualty in taking one aspirin tablet (300mg) which could slow the clotting process down by thinning the blood.
>
> However, some people are allergic to aspirin and it could have a detrimental effect on them.
>
> If you are unsure about the allergy, then DO NOT administer it.
>
> You must not administer an aspirin to anyone under the age of 16, and it should not be kept in the first aid kit.

STROKE

In simplistic terms, a stroke is a brain attack. A stroke is a serious medical condition that occurs when the blood supply to part of the brain is cut off.

Like all organs, the brain needs the oxygen and nutrients provided by blood to function properly. If the supply of blood is restricted or stopped, brain cells begin to die. This can lead to brain damage and possibly death.

Strokes are a medical emergency and prompt treatment is essential because the sooner your casualty receives treatment for a stroke, the less damage is likely to happen to them.

Types of stroke
There are two main causes of strokes:

- **Ischaemic** (accounting for over 80% of all cases): **the blood supply is stopped due to a blood clot**
- **Haemorrhagic: a weakened blood vessel supplying the brain bursts and causes brain damage**

There is also a related condition known as a **transient ischaemic attack (TIA)**, where the supply of blood to the brain is temporarily interrupted, causing a 'mini-stroke'. TIA's should be treated as being serious as they are often a warning sign that a stroke is coming.

Strokes can damage:

- **Bodily functions**
- **Our thought processes**
- **Our ability to learn**
- **How we feel and communicate**

If you suspect a stroke – act **FAST** and call 999/112 for an ambulance.

Treatment

- **If the casualty is responsive, lay them down and raise their head and shoulders**
- **Turn their head to one side, affected side down**
- **If the casualty is unresponsive, place them in the recovery position injured side down**
- **Loosen tight clothing**
- **Reassure them and call for an ambulance**
- **Monitor their airway, breathing and response levels. Be prepared to resuscitate them**

Stroke is a medical emergency.

By calling for an ambulance early, treatment can be given which can prevent further brain damage.

F Facial weakness

Can the person smile?
Has their mouth or eye drooped?

A Arm weakness

Can the person raise both arms?

S Speech problems

Can the person speak clearly and understand what you say?

T Time to call 999/112

MAJOR ILLNESSES continued

DIABETES

Diabetes is a long-term condition caused by too much glucose, a type of sugar, in the blood. It is also known as diabetes mellitus.

Normally, the amount of sugar in the blood is controlled by a hormone called insulin. Insulin is produced by the pancreas, a gland located behind the stomach. When food is digested and enters the bloodstream, insulin helps move any glucose out of the blood and into cells, where it is broken down to produce energy.

For people with diabetes, the body is unable to break down glucose into energy. This is because there is either not enough insulin to move the glucose, or because the insulin that is there does not work properly.

There are two types of diabetes: type 1 and type 2 diabetes.

Type 1 diabetes occurs when the body produces no insulin. It is often referred to as insulin-dependent diabetes. It is also sometimes known as juvenile diabetes or early-onset diabetes because it usually develops before the age of 40, often during the teenage years.

Type 2 diabetes occurs when not enough insulin is produced by the body for it to function properly, or when the body's cells do not react to insulin. This is called insulin resistance.
It is far more common than type 1.
Around 90% of all adults in the UK with diabetes have type 2.

General signs and symptoms
- **Feeling very thirsty**
- **Going to the toilet a lot, especially at night**
- **Extreme tiredness**
- **Weight loss and muscle wasting**
  (loss of muscle bulk)

Hyperglycaemia occurs when there is a higher than normal level of glucose (sugar) in the blood.

This causes:
- **Increased thirst**
- **The need to urinate frequently**
- **Tiredness**

Hypoglycaemia means that there is an abnormally low level of sugar (glucose) in the blood.

When the glucose level is too low – called a 'hypo' – the body does not have enough energy to carry out its activities.

Most people will have some warning that their blood glucose levels are too low, which will give them time to correct it.

Typical early warning signs are:
- **Feeling hungry**
- **Trembling or shakiness**
- **Sweating**

Treatment
Hyperglycaemia
- Call for an ambulance
- If they become unresponsive, place them in the recovery position
- Monitor their breathing and response levels

Treatment
Hypoglycaemia
- Sit the casualty down
- Offer them 15-20gms of glucose. Offer a sugary drink or sweet food if glucose is not available
- Monitor and reassure them
- Call for an ambulance if the above is ineffective
- If they become unresponsive, place them in the recovery position and monitor them

	HYPERglycaemia	HYPOglycaemia
Amount of insulin used	Not enough	Too much
Deterioration	Gradual	Very quick
Hunger	Absent	Present
Vomiting	Common	Uncommon
Thirst	Present	Absent
Breath odour	Fruity/sweet	Normal
Pulse	Rapid and weak	Rapid
Breathing	Rapid	Normal
Skin	Dry and warm	Pale, cold and sweaty
Seizures	Uncommon	Common
Responsiveness	Drowsy	Rapid loss

ASTHMA

Asthma is caused by an inflammation to the airways, and in particular the small tubes, called bronchi, which carry air in and out of the lungs. For those who have asthma, the bronchi will be inflamed and more sensitive than normal. When they come into contact with something that irritates their lungs, known as a trigger, their airways become narrow, the muscles around them tighten and there is an increase in the production of sticky mucus (phlegm).

This makes it difficult to breathe and causes wheezing and coughing. It may also make their chest feel tight.

A severe onset of symptoms is known as an asthma attack. Asthma attacks may require hospital treatment and can sometimes be life-threatening, although this is rare.

For some people with chronic (long-lasting) asthma, long-term inflammation of the airways may lead to more permanent narrowing.

Signs and symptoms
- Difficulty in breathing
- Wheezing
- Distress and anxiety
- Difficulty in speaking
- Grey/blue skin tones
- May become exhausted
- Coughing

Treatment
- Alleviate their concerns by calming them and offering plenty of support and reassurance
- Make them comfortable and relaxed by sitting them down
- Allow them to use their own inhaler

Dial 999/112 if:
- The medication has no effect after 5 minutes
- If it's the first attack
- Breathlessness makes talking difficult

EFFECTS OF EXTREME HEAT AND COLD

HYPOTHERMIA

Hypothermia occurs when a person's normal body temperature of around 37°C (98.6°F) drops below 35°C (95°F).

It is usually caused by being in a cold environment. It can be triggered by a combination of things, including prolonged exposure to cold (such as staying outdoors in cold conditions or in a poorly heated room for a long time), rain, wind, sweat, inactivity or being in cold water.

Signs and symptoms

The symptoms of hypothermia depend on how cold the environment is and how long your casualty is exposed for.

Severe hypothermia needs urgent medical treatment in hospital. Shivering is a good guide to how severe the condition is. If the person can stop shivering on their own, the hypothermia is mild, but if they cannot stop shivering, it is moderate to severe.

MILD CASES

In mild cases, symptoms include:

- Shivering
- Feeling cold
- Low energy
- Cold, pale skin

MODERATE CASES

The symptoms of moderate hypothermia include:

- Violent, uncontrollable shivering
- Being unable to think or pay attention
- Confusion (some people don't realise they are affected)
- Loss of judgement and reasoning
- Difficulty moving around or stumbling (weakness)
- Feeling afraid
- Memory loss
- Fumbling hands and loss of coordination
- Drowsiness
- Slurred speech
- Listlessness and indifferent
- Slow, shallow breathing and a weak pulse

SEVERE CASES

The symptoms of severe hypothermia include:

- Loss of control of hands, feet, and limbs
- Uncontrollable shivering that suddenly stops
- Unresponsiveness
- Shallow or no breathing
- Weak, irregular or no pulse
- Stiff muscles
- Dilated pupils

Treating hypothermia

As hypothermia can be a life-threatening condition, seek medical attention as soon as possible.

Hypothermia is treated by preventing further heat being lost and by gently warming the casualty.

If you are treating someone with mild hypothermia at home, or waiting for medical treatment to arrive, follow the advice below to prevent further loss of heat.

- Move the casualty indoors, or somewhere warm, as soon as possible
- Once sheltered, gently remove any wet clothing and dry them
- Wrap them in blankets, towels, coats (whatever you have), protecting the head and torso first
- Increase activity if possible, but not to the point where sweating occurs, as that cools the skin down again
- If possible, give them warm drinks (but not alcohol) or high energy foods, such as chocolate, to help warm them up
- Once their body temperature has increased, keep them warm and dry

It is important to handle anyone that has hypothermia very gently and carefully.

Things you should NOT do:

- **Do not warm up an elderly person using a bath**, as this may send cold blood from the body's surfaces to the heart or brain too suddenly, causing a stroke or heart attack
- **Do not apply direct heat** (hot water or a heating pad, for example) to the arms and legs, as this forces cold blood back to the major organs, making the condition worse
- **Do not give them alcohol to drink**, as this will decrease the body's ability to retain heat
- **Do not rub or massage their skin**, as this can cause the blood vessels to widen and decrease the body's ability to retain heat. In severe cases of hypothermia there is also a risk of heart attack

---

When to seek medical help

If someone you know has been exposed to the cold and they're distressed or confused, and they have slow, shallow breathing or they're unresponsive, they may have severe hypothermia. Their skin may look healthy but feel cold. Babies may also be limp, unusually quiet and refuse to feed.

Cases of severe hypothermia require urgent medical treatment in hospital. You should call 999 to request an ambulance if you suspect that someone you know has severe hypothermia. Do not give them any food or drink.

As the body temperature drops, shivering will stop completely. The heart rate will slow and your casualty will gradually lose responsiveness.

Be prepared to resuscitate if they stop breathing normally.

FIRST AID AT WORK

HEAT EXHAUSTION

Heat exhaustion is brought on when the temperature inside the body, known as the core temperature, rises from the normal 37°C up to 40°C (98.6 – 104°F). At that temperature, the levels of water and salt in the body begin to drop. This causes symptoms such as nausea, feeling faint and heavy sweating.

If it is left untreated, heat exhaustion can sometimes lead to heatstroke.

Signs and symptoms
- Pale, clammy skin
- Heavy sweating
- Dizziness
- Fatigue
- Nausea
- Vomiting
- Rapid heartbeat
- Mental confusion
- Urinating less often and the colour of the urine being much darker than usual

Treatment
- **Get them to rest in a cool place,** ideally in a room with air conditioning, or at least somewhere that is in the shade
- **Give them plenty of fluids to drink.** This should either be water or a rehydration drink such as a sports drink. Avoid alcohol or caffeine as this can increase dehydration
- **Cool their skin with cold water.** If available, use a shower or cold bath to cool them down. If not, then apply wet towels to their skin
- **Loosen any unnecessary clothing,** and make sure that the person gets plenty of air

HEATSTROKE

Heatstroke happens when a person's core temperature rises above 40°C (104°F). Cells inside the body begin to break down and important parts of the body stop working.

Heatstroke is a medical emergency. If left untreated, it can cause multiple organ failure, brain damage and death.

Signs and symptoms
- **High body temperature:** having a temperature of 40°C (104°F) or above is a major sign of heatstroke
- Hot and dry skin
- Not sweating even while feeling too hot
- Rapid heartbeat
- Rapid breathing
- Muscle cramps

Treatment
- Move the casualty to a cool area as quickly as possible
- Increase the air supply by opening windows or using a fan
- Give them water to drink if possible, but do not give them any medication
- Shower the skin with cool, but not cold, water (15°C-18°C). If there is no shower nearby, cover the body with cool, damp towels or sheets, or immerse in cool water
- If any of the muscles are cramped, gently massage the skin to encourage circulation
- If seizures start, move nearby objects out of the way to prevent injury (do not use force or put anything in the mouth)
- If the casualty is unresponsive and vomiting, place them in the recovery position
- Call 999/112 for an ambulance

SECTION 25 | PAGE 57

BITES AND STINGS

Animal and human bites are a relatively common type of injury. In most cases, the wound that results from an animal bite is minor and can be treated with simple first aid techniques.

DOG BITES

Dog bites typically cause a puncture wound (a narrow and deep hole) in the skin. They can also cause a laceration (a jagged wound or cut) and an abrasion (a scraped area of skin).

This is because dogs use their front teeth to "pin" their victim, and their other teeth to bite and pull at the surrounding skin.

CAT BITES

A cat bite is not as strong as a dog's, but their teeth are sharper and often cause very deep puncture wounds. A cat bite is capable of penetrating bones and joints. Lacerations and abrasions are less common, occurring in one-in-five cases.

HUMAN BITES

Most human bites are the result of a closed-fist injury, where one person punches another person in the teeth and cuts their hand. Typical symptoms include small cuts to the hand, and red, swollen and painful skin.

Toddlers often bite each other when playing together, but the resulting injuries are usually minor and do not usually pose a serious risk to their health.

General treatment
- Make the area safe
- Reduce the risk of infection by wearing gloves
- Clean the wound immediately by running warm tap water over it for a couple of minutes
- Inspect the wound for embedded objects such as teeth and remove if you are able to
- Dry the wound and cover it with a sterile dressing
- Treat for shock

When to seek medical advice:

You should seek immediate medical attention for all but minor dog or cat bites.

However, even some minor-looking cat bites can penetrate deeply and become infected.

Human bites have a much higher chance of causing infection, so always seek immediate medical attention before waiting for any symptoms of infection to appear.

Symptoms of infection
- **Redness and swelling around the wound.** The wound becomes more painful
- **Discharge from the wound**
- **Swollen lymph glands** (nodes)
- **A high temperature** (fever) **of 38°C** (100.4°F) **or above**
- **Shivers**

Always seek immediate medical attention if you or your child receives a bite to the following areas:
- The hands
- The feet
- A joint, tendon or ligament
- The scalp or face
- The genitals
- The ears or nose

Dial 999 immediately to request an ambulance if your child receives bite wounds to their head, neck or face. These types of wound can cause high amounts of blood loss, particularly in young children aged 10 or under and babies, and may therefore require emergency treatment.

If they have been bitten, the most important thing to do is to clean the wound immediately by running run warm tap water over the wound for 10 minutes.

In cases of serious bites, where a body part such as a finger or ear has been bitten off, you should wash the body part with tap water and place it in a plastic bag or a sealed container. Put the bag or container into a tub of iced water (but not frozen) to keep it cool, so that it can be transported to hospital. It may be possible to reattach the body part using reconstructive surgery.